FIT
OVER FORTY

Previous books by James M. Rippe, M.D.

The Exercise Exchange Program

The Complete Book of Fitness Walking

Fit for Success

The Rockport Walking Program

Fitness Walking for Women

The Sports Performance Factors

Fitness Walking

FIT
OVER FORTY

A REVOLUTIONARY PLAN TO ACHIEVE LIFELONG

PHYSICAL AND SPIRITUAL HEALTH AND WELL-BEING

JAMES M. RIPPE, M.D.

QUILL

WILLIAM MORROW

NEW YORK

It is the policy of William Morrow and Company, Inc., and its imprints and affiliates, recognizing the importance of preserving what has been written, to print the books we publish on acid-free paper, and we exert our best efforts to that end.

Library of Congress Cataloging-in-Publication Data

Rippe, James M.
    Fit over forty : a revolutionary plan to achieve lifelong physical and spiritual health and well-being / James M. Rippe, M.D.
        p.   cm.
    Includes bibliographical references and index.
    ISBN 0-688-15399-2
    1. Middle aged persons—Health and hygiene.   2. Physical fitness for the aged.
    3. Physical fitness—Religious aspects.   4. Middle aged persons—Religious life.
    I. Title.
    RA777.5.R57   1996
    613'.0434—dc20

                                                                        96-6844
                                                                        CIP

Printed in the United States of America

First Quill Edition

            5   6   7   8   9   10

BOOK DESIGN BY MICHAEL MENDELSOHN OF MM DESIGN 2000, INC.

To
Stephanie,
who gave me
Hart

AUTHOR'S NOTE

The final shape and clarity of this book are a tribute to Mary Abbott Waite. Mary Abbott is every writer's dream collaborator. She took a long, heartfelt, but sometimes rambling manuscript and sculpted it into a more focused, streamlined, and logical book. Along the way she added numerous insights, personal touches, and pearls of wisdom drawn from her deep commitment and experiences as a fellow traveler on the "over forty road to fitness." Without her friendship, intelligence, calm competence, and editorial skills, this book would not have been possible.

FOREWORDS

When I was ten years old and playing ball with a bunch of friends, I never dreamed I'd be playing in the majors, let alone playing baseball into my forties. As a kid, I had no concept of physical conditioning; I just knew I liked to throw the ball. But the longer I played, the more I realized how important physical conditioning is. I know now that if I hadn't been so committed to fitness, I never could have stayed in the game so long.

That's why I've teamed up with Dr. James Rippe, Peggy Fleming, and the Advil Forum on Health Education to get the message out about the importance of fitness and the benefits of the Advil Fit over Forty Standards. Now that my career doesn't depend on physical conditioning, I'm finding it challenging to find time to exercise. And I'm as guilty as anyone of putting it off until tomorrow.

What's the secret? There really is no secret to staying fit. But there are a lot of misconceptions—including the idea that physical activity takes too much time.

This book is designed to help. By charting your progress with Advil Fit over Forty Standards and incorporating some of Dr. Rippe's simple health tips into your lifestyle, you will see how easy physical fitness can be. The fact is: You don't need lots of time to commit to fitness, and it's never too late to get started.

My wife, Ruth, and I think that staying fit should be fun and enjoyable, and that's what we've tried to teach our kids, Reid, Reese, and Wendy. We make it something we look forward to, rather than dread. We walk together, play tennis, run with the dogs, play ball with our kids . . . being active has become such an integral part of our lives that it's never a chore.

There's no question that being more physically fit is one of the best things you can do to improve your health. I hope this book will help you accomplish all of your fitness goals.

Good luck!

—NOLAN RYAN

Physical activity has always been important to me. In fact, I can still remember my delight at being able to run the fastest or hit a ball farther than the other children. As a little girl, I loved any sport or game that challenged my coordination and strength, and as a woman today I am much the same. Exercise and physical challenge have not only shaped my life, they've defined much of who I am.

Ironically, my first memory of stepping onto the ice at age nine is not one of challenge but one of quite effortless movement. The years that followed that first day were full of long practices, tedious figures, and extreme dedication. But the joy of movement is the memory that has always stayed the strongest.

Since winning the Olympic Gold Medal in 1968, my skating has earned me a place in the U.S. Olympic Hall of Fame and the Women's Sports Foundation Hall of Fame. I am extremely honored by this recognition and feel very lucky to have found a sport that has inspired my spirit as well as my body. I also realize that none of this would have been possible without a dedication to fitness.

That's why I'm so pleased to be working with Dr. Rippe, Nolan Ryan, and the Advil Forum on Health Education. We all believe strongly in making exercise an important part of life, for ourselves and our families, and want to share our enthusiasm about fitness. Being fit takes dedication, but the benefits are tremendous.

It really is never too late to begin.

—PEGGY FLEMING

ACKNOWLEDGMENTS

Research, patient care, and book writing are all collaborative efforts. Over the years, I have been blessed with incredible friends and colleagues in all these areas, to whom I am deeply grateful.

The research project that resulted in The Advil Fit over Forty Standards, the cornerstone body of scientific work behind this book, was conducted by a tireless and dedicated group of researchers in my laboratory. Researchers making major contributions included: Chris Palmer, M.S., Stacey Hess, M.S., Susanne Damitz, R.N., M.S., Kimberly DeMers, R.D., Keith DeRuisseau, B.S., Imad Kreidieh, M.D., and Janet Price, M.D. My long-term friend and research associate Patty Freedson, Ph.D., contributed insights and constructive comments throughout the project. Gregory Kline, Ph.D., provided the overall statistical plan and supervised the final analyses.

While this research team conducted the final project to establish the first-ever comprehensive fitness standards for individuals over the age of forty, many other talented researchers have contributed to studies from my laboratory which are cited throughout this book. Some of those who have made particularly important contributions include: Ann Ward, Ph.D., Lynn Ahlquist, Ph.D., Cara Ebbeling, M.S., Pamela Taylor, M.D., Daniel Carlucci, M.D., Bonita Marks, Ph.D., Edith Fletcher, R.N., David Brown, Ph.D., Youde Wang, Ph.D., Diane Morris, Ph.D., R.D., John Castellani, M.S., John Porcari, Ph.D., Jeff Widrick, Ph.D., Merry Yamartino, R.D., Laurie Fortlage, R.D., Elaine Puleo, Ph.D., Christine Ebbeling, M.S., Sadri Ahmadi, M.S., Stephanie O'Hanley, M.S., and Robert Hintermeister, Ph.D.

Friends, professional colleagues, and mentors have helped at various stages in my life and professional development. Often they have strengthened my convictions and clarified my thinking both as a researcher and as a physician. John McCarthy, executive director of International Health and Racquets Sports Association, has been a long-term supporter of our work and has helped guide my thinking about the links between fitness and health. Augie Nieto and Bob Hood, president and executive vice president of Life Fitness respectively, have been instrumental in many of the research projects that yielded information for this book. Richard Boggs, president of The STEP Company, has been and remains an important friend and adviser. Linda Webb Carilli, M.S., R.D., director of communications of Weight Watchers International, and Florine Mark, president and CEO of the Weight Watchers Group, have lent valuable insights into issues related to healthy weight management. Tony Harmon, president of Polar Electro, Inc., has supported and refined our work on various aspects of heart-rate monitoring related to stress reduction and exercise.

Ruth Stricker and Bruce Dayton have been long-term friends and supporters of the Center for Clinical and Lifestyle Research and mentors in the area of mind/body interactions. Joe Beckwith, senior vice president of McDonald's, is a friend and colleague who has helped me understand vision and leadership, particularly as fitness applies to the needs of children and families. Kathy Hartman, vice president of marketing for Discovery Zone, has also helped me understand issues related to families and children. Ginna Frantz, president of V.M. Frantz and Company, has been a long-term friend and colleague who has helped me learn how to better communicate complex messages related to health and fitness.

My colleagues at the Television Food Network (TVFN) have taught me a great deal about how to communicate health, fitness, and nutrition messages to the public. Reese Shoenfeld, the founding CEO of TVFN, gave me the confidence to believe that I could effectively communicate on television. Donna Hanover, anchorwoman at TVFN and first lady of New York City, and David Rosengarten, co-anchor at TVFN, have been friends and mentors in the area of electronic communication. Dr. Lou Aronne and Gayle Gardner, co-hosts of *Getting Healthy*, have been friends and important colleagues. Richard Leibner, my television agent, has been a constant source of creative ideas and constructive input.

My first mentor in medicine, Dr. Joseph Alpert, taught me that a physician's personality and kindness are as important as medical facts in the treatment of patients. Dr. Ira Ockene continued my education as a cardiologist and has been a long-term friend and teacher. Dr. Richard Irwin has been my colleague and co-editor of *Intensive Care Medicine* and a long-term friend and supporter. Dr. Mike Fox has been a friend and confidant and a steady source of advice about various personal and professional issues. Dr. John Harrington, acting dean at Tufts University School of Medicine, has supported my ongoing development as both a physician and medical communicator.

I am very grateful to my literary agent, Reid Boates, who believed so strongly in this project and made the connections between William Morrow, Mary Abbott Waite, and me. My editor at William Morrow, Henry Ferris, has been a wonderful friend and endless source of energy, enthusiasm, and creativity throughout the entire book-writing project.

Many individuals at American Home Products and its subsidiary, Whitehall-Robins, the makers of Advil, have supported the research work behind this project and been great believers in this book. Without their support, the research project that underlies this book would not have been possible.

My hardworking and creative friends at Edelman Public Relations have been a constant source of encouragement and support throughout the entire book-writing project and during the research project that led up to it. Lisa Sepulveda, senior vice president, was one of the great early advocates of this project and has continued to be a source both of wisdom and energy. Sheila Marmion, vice president, Bronwyn Fenton, senior account supervisor, and Debbie Yerman Lobel, account supervisor, have also been great proponents and contributors to the project. Richard Edelman, president and Co-CEO, was an early backer, and remains an ardent supporter of the whole concept of getting people over the age of forty to be more fit and healthy.

I am grateful to my friends Nolan Ryan and Peggy Fleming for agreeing to write Forewords to this book. Both have been enormously supportive of the book's concept and both epitomize in their personal lives the multiple benefits of lifelong fitness. Nolan has also been my friend and companion on travels around the country promoting the concept that every person can be more fit and healthy as the result of simple daily practices and decisions.

The great physician Sir William Osler once said that to study medicine without books would be to go to sea without a ship but to study medicine without patients would be never to put to sea at all. Certainly I am deeply grateful to all the patients and research subjects who contributed in so many ways to this book. I am thankful to the 349 subjects who gave so generously of their time, energy, and insight during the yearlong research project to establish The Advil Fit over Forty Standards. I am also grateful to the many thousands of research subjects and patients whom I have cared for, and learned from, over the past twenty years. In one way or another, all of them have contributed to the content, shape, and direction of this book. Throughout this manuscript, names have been changed and in some instances experiences condensed to illustrate points and protect anonymity.

No project of this magnitude would be possible without my superb editorial and support staff. Elizabeth Porcaro has been my editorial assistant for over twelve years. Her great organizational skills, boundless energy, and commitment to me and all of my diverse projects remain a great source of joy and pride to me. No project of the scope of this book or any of my other numerous publishing projects would be possible without Beth's wonderful efforts.

My executive assistant, Carol Moreau, manages an extremely complex consulting, speaking, and traveling schedule with grace and good humor. She manages to find ways to carve out the time so necessary for the complex task of writing. Previous executive assistants Janet LaBonte and Sherri Herland also did a wonderful job of assisting me during various phases of this and previous research projects and books.

My family continues to be a source of great comfort and support to me. My brothers, Dr. Richard Rippe and Dr. William Rippe, and their wives, Sandy and Marcia, and their children have all wrapped me in their love.

Finally, to my dear wife, Stephanie, whom I owe a special debt of gratitude. Stephanie has lifted me and cradled me in her love, helped me stop and smell the roses, and given me the strength and courage to pursue the dreams outlined in the book.

—J.M.R.
Boston, Massachusetts

CONTENTS

PART ONE: FIT OVER FORTY

PART TWO: TOWARD A FITTER LIFESTYLE

PART THREE: FIT OVER FORTY FITNESS PROGRAMS

PART ONE

FIT
OVER FORTY

CHAPTER 1

FIT OVER FORTY: A NEW APPROACH TO FITNESS

THE JOURNEY

This is a book about hope and a new vision of health and fitness.

This is a book about feeling good—better than you ever have, better than you ever thought possible. It is also a book about the personal power to be healthier than you've ever been by paying attention to daily practices and habits. It is a book about mind and body, a plan for achieving physical health and spiritual well-being.

This is a book about groundbreaking science. It is based on a landmark study conducted in my laboratory that established, for the first time ever, comprehensive fitness standards for people over the age of forty, The Advil Fit over Forty Standards. These standards enable us for the first time to establish what it really means to be fit at each decade of life. The book also draws on ten years of studies in my exercise and nutrition laboratory and many others that have reshaped our understanding of health and fitness.

This is a book about shattering old concepts and building new models of what you must do to be fit and healthy. Based on new views of health and fitness, the book offers a set of simple home tests to enable you to evaluate your overall fitness profile. It then provides complete programs in every component area of fitness so that you can design your own plan for achieving optimal health and improved fitness.

This is a book about simplicity. None of the steps you must take to develop positive daily habits and practices is complex or difficult.

This is, most important of all, a book about a journey and about bridges. The journey is yours, mine, everyone's. When we are young, most of us take health and fitness for granted as we focus on building our lives. But by the time we hit forty, most of us have experienced hints of mortality. We begin to pay attention. None of us wants to be "old" before our "time." In fact, we reject the concept of aging as "deteriorating." We want to live life fully every step of the way. Providing a road map and the bridges to reach that goal is the purpose of this book.

As guide and fellow over-forty traveler I invite you to take a journey with me toward this goal of living fully and healthfully. During my twenty years in medicine I have had the opportunity to care for thousands of patients, and in my research laboratory we've had the opportunity to study (and learn from) thousands more. Along the way I have learned a lot about how to help people help themselves. Some of the things I've learned may surprise you. But I also think they will please you. The scientific and medical discoveries in fitness and health over the past decade have been truly astounding. Most important, they have confirmed what many believed and hoped for all along: that our bodies have innate wisdom and healing power, that living fully, consciously, and healthfully is also living simply.

But this is more than a professional journey for me, it is also a highly personal one. In writing the book for every person over forty who wants to live fully and healthfully, I am writing it for myself. The scientific principles and the fitness programs shared in this book have not just been proved in my laboratory and others; I have experienced their effectiveness in my life and in the lives of my patients.

I started to study medicine twenty years ago with the conviction that health was a great value and that each of us could be healthier through our own efforts. While some aspects of this belief have undergone subtle changes, the basic conviction remains. We now have the research and the techniques to support this conviction. If you want to feel healthier and happier than you ever thought possible, I'm going to ask you to make some changes, but they will be simple ones—surprisingly simple. And this book will provide the bridges you need to make this journey to a new lifestyle. Let's look at them.

BRIDGES

The biggest problem in getting started on a fitness program is not lack of knowing that we need to do something but bridging the chasm between intention and action. Survey after survey has shown that over 90 percent of adults agree that their daily habits have an impact on their long-term health. In a recent survey published in *USA Today*, for example, 93 percent of the respondents agreed that regular exercise was one of the best habits each of us could adopt to preserve or enhance our health. Yet many studies show that less than 20 percent of us are active on a regular basis.

In my experience, most people have trouble acting on health-promoting measures because they make them too complex. Often people suffer from the misconception that they need to turn their lives upside down to be healthier. Nothing could be further from the truth. In fact, it is the accumulation of small, simple adjustments in our daily habits and practices that make the long-term difference. In this book I am going to show you how to make those simple adjustments that will change your life forever and for the better. Here are the three important tools we'll use to help you bridge the chasm between intention and action:

The Advil Fit over Forty Standards

Introduced in their entirety in this book, these provide comprehensive measures by which we can determine what it means to be fit at each decade of life. Until this study such standards had never been available. Now they enable us to evaluate what realistic goals can be set in many component areas of fitness: cardiovascular fitness, strength (muscular fitness), flexibility, balance, mobility, stress, nutrition, weight management.

The Fit over Forty Fitness Profile Tests

Developed on and tested for individuals over the age of forty, these ten home tests provide an easy, safe, and accurate way to access your overall fitness levels. By using the Advil Fit over Forty Standards and these tests to develop a Personal Fitness Profile, individuals over forty will be able, for the first time, to compare their results with those of others of the same age and sex and to use the results to get started on safe and effective programs to improve their health and fitness forever.

The Fit over Forty Fitness Programs

Knowledge is power—if you put it into action. This book provides specific fitness programs in each of the component areas tested so that once you've identified where you need to work, you can get started right away. All these activity programs have been used extensively by patients at my clinics. We know they work.

In addition to these specific programs, I'll be sharing many insights into the role that being physically active, paying attention to mind-body interactions, and striving for functional fitness can play in helping you move toward a fitter lifestyle. I'll also share some special recommendations about relating our goals of fitness to issues of aging and special health considerations.

TOWARD A NEW VISION OF FITNESS

A moment ago I invited you to join me on a journey toward fitness and fulfillment. It is going to be an exciting journey, which will take us to places different from those you might imagine. As you'll see, fitness is not just about exercise, although that is certainly a part of it. Fitness is about life and joy and peace. Fitness is about rising to meet the challenges that each of us faces every day. It is about discovering the power that lies within us to live happier, fuller, and healthier lives than we ever thought possible. It is about listening to the healer who lives inside each of us. It is a journey to the center of our being. It is a journey to discover not just who we are but who we can be. I invite you to start the journey by going on to the next chapter, as we consider more fully what it means to be fit.

CHAPTER 2

WHAT DOES IT MEAN TO BE FIT?

MARK

In his mid-forties Mark had risen to be vice-president of sales of a large manufacturing company. Hard-living and fast-talking, he was a smart salesman who could sell you almost anything his company manufactured and convince you to be grateful for the opportunity to purchase it (whether you needed it or not).

For a smart guy, he was also plenty reckless with his health. He smoked cigarettes, paid virtually no attention to his diet, and spent most days sitting in his car or at meetings. Not surprisingly, his weight had crept up thirty-five pounds in the two decades since college.

At the age of forty-eight Mark had a heart attack.

When I first met him in my office three weeks following the heart attack, he was plainly shaken. But he also felt lucky because he was still alive. The statistics, so familiar to me, had been drummed into him during his ten-day hospital stay: Half of all people who suffer heart attacks die before they make it to the hospital.

To make a long (and wonderfully inspiring) story short, Mark's heart attack served as a major wake-up call. He decided to stop, look, listen—and get his life in order. He made a commitment to reclaim a life that had been spinning out of control. He stopped smoking. It was hard, but he crumpled up his last pack of cigarettes and threw it away.

He starting lowering the fat in his regular diet—at first because I told him he had to and later because he felt so much better that he couldn't imagine eating the way he used to. He started a daily walking program that ultimately progressed to a walk-jog program. Over the next two years the thirty-five pounds he had gained since college slowly melted away. He looked and felt better than he ever had before—ever!

I actually used to run into Mark from time to time outside our office visits since our walking and running routes intersected at a few spots. After a particularly great jog one day Mark told me a story I've never forgotten.

It seems that a number of his salesmen buddies had been chiding him about his newfound commitment to health and fitness. One had accused Mark's new program of turning him into a narcissist.

"At first it really made me mad," Mark said, "but as I thought about it, I decided maybe I *am* a narcissist, in the sense that I have come to love myself, my body and my health. You know, it reminded me of my father. He had all the same habits that I had before my heart attack. He smoked too much, ate high fat foods, never exercised, and worried about work incessantly."

Mark paused and looked at me. "At the age of forty-five he dropped dead in our family's kitchen of a massive heart attack. Maybe I am a narcissist. Maybe if my father had loved himself more, he would have taken better care of himself and not left my mother with three young children to raise by herself."

Just what does it mean to be fit? Whether or not we've had wake-up calls as dramatic as Mark's (and most of us haven't), we all want to be fit and healthy. But we are not sure just what that means—either in general or for ourselves individually. Each day's news seems to bring new studies and new advice, often seemingly contradictory. The whole issue seems too complex to understand, much less to act on. And most of us don't. More than 80 percent of adult Americans don't exercise regularly; 40 percent are entirely sedentary. Our primary excuse? Not enough time.

These facts are why I'm convinced that a new vision of fitness is so important as a starting place. Based on the burgeoning scientific research of the last few years, this new understanding is grounded in the one important thing that we all can learn from Mark's experience:

Learning to love yourself enough to value your physical health and emotional/spiritual well-being is the foundation of living fully and happily.

During my work with thousands of patients and research subjects, I've come to agree with what Thornton Wilder says at the end of *The Bridge of San Luis Rey*, that there truly is "a land of the living and a land of the dead." And the bridge that takes you into the land of the living is the bridge you build, just as Mark did, when you claim a new vision of what living fully means.

PROSPERITY AND PEACE: A NEW VISION OF FITNESS

During a recent presidential election campaign a political analyst declared that despite the many issues dividing the candidates, the only issues that really mattered to the public were prosperity and peace. While any generalization risks oversimplifying, I think this journalist was generally right: All of us want to believe that we are basically doing all right and have achieved a measure of personal and economic security, but at the same time each of us desires meaning and tranquillity.

Unfortunately a lot of us have forgotten that prosperity and peace are strongly linked in our personal lives. Just look back at the go-go 1980s. With a rapidly expanding economy many people thought that prosperity was a given and would last forever. We pursued material gains and measured self-worth by the size of our houses or stock portfolios or the types of car we drove. In a strange way, our approach to fitness mirrored these larger trends. There was an almost fanatical determination behind many people's exercise routines as they sought personal records, tight abdominal muscles, and low body fat. "No pain, no gain" and "Go for the burn!" were the mantras of the day (two notions that have certainly done more harm than good).

Then the bubble burst. The stock market fell more than five hundred points in one day. Companies started to downsize, throwing people out of work for the first time in their lives. People found themselves sore and sad in their fitness programs or, worse, fat and unhappy, sitting on the sidelines, having failed once again to establish a reasonable plan for long-term fitness.

Most important, we all got older. The entire population grayed. In

1988, for the first time in our country's history, the number of people over the age of forty exceeded those below the age of thirty. And as we got older, we began to see what happens when we lose our way. We got stressed out, inactive, and fat. We began to see our loved ones who hadn't taken care of themselves get sick and die. We began to experience our own mortality. For all these reasons, and many more, as the 1990s dawned, many people began to look around and say, "Is that all there is?"

My response to that question is a resounding "No! There's much more!"

By pursuing "prosperity" in all aspects of our lives, whether through accumulating material goods or chasing a grim-faced, hard-edged fitness, many of us lost our way. What we need is a new vision of health and fitness, one that is more consistent with the realities of our lives, one that we can enjoy and stick with, and, yes, one that is based on solid scientific and medical information. Fortunately, while we were locked into our quest for hard bodies and material goods, the scientific underpinnings of a new vision of health and fitness began to emerge.

- Do you want to save your heart? Take a pleasant walk.
- Stressed out? Take ten minutes each day to listen to your heart.
- Tired of those pulled muscles? Get strong.
- Want to function at your peak? Stay active.
- Want to lower your risk of cancer? Eat more fruits and vegetables.

My point is that simple things, things we often overlook, have the power to heal us. This is the greatest lesson that I have learned from science and from personal and professional experience in twenty years of medical practice. Sharing a bit of my journey of discovery will help you understand more fully what this new approach can mean for you.

A PERSONAL AND SCIENTIFIC JOURNEY TOWARD A NEW UNDERSTANDING OF FITNESS

Like many others in the late sixties and early seventies, I was an avid, even obsessional jogger. By the time, at age twenty-seven, I entered Harvard Medical School I was running some serious distances—often forty to fifty miles per week. Even at those distances I wondered if I was doing enough. After all, according to the fitness ideas of the time, if some was good, then more must be better! I had little idea then that "going for the burn" and those additional miles weren't helping my health and might even be damaging it.

With running as my serious hobby, it wasn't surprising that when we started to study the cardiovascular system I immediately found my calling. Becoming a cardiologist was the perfect way to combine business with pleasure. And since our nation was undergoing an epidemic of cardiovascular disease in the 1970s (an epidemic that continues to this day), entering the field of cardiovascular medicine also seemed a perfect way to contribute to the solution to the number one health problem facing our country.

By the time I finished my training and joined the faculty at the University of Massachusetts Medical School, I was well versed in the most advanced medical and surgical techniques for treating coronary disease. About this time the results of important trials in the *prevention* of cardiovascular disease were also beginning to be published. The Framingham Heart Study had established clear-cut risk factors for heart disease, such as cigarette smoking, elevated cholesterol, and high blood pressure. Dr. Ralph Paffenbarger had begun to publish the results of his College Alumni Study showing that inactivity presented a significant risk for coronary heart disease.

While I knew about these studies, I, like most cardiologists, relied heavily on high tech medicine. I treated desperately ill heart attack patients in the coronary care unit and performed cardiac catheterizations in the high tech atmosphere of a university cardiac catheterization laboratory. I believed that if people wouldn't take care of their own coronary arteries, then at least we could fix them with such techniques as coronary artery bypass grafting and angioplasty.

It took me several years and several thousand cardiac catheterizations before I began to put things in perspective. Often in the cardiac catheterization laboratory I saw myself as a farmer standing at an open barn door desperately grasping for the tail of a horse as it bolted out of the barn. This was what we were doing with our patients. We were trying valiantly to help them after the horse was already out of the barn. There had to be a better way. We had to find a way to keep the barn door closed.

Fortunately two counterweights were pulling me in the opposite direction. The first was my patient practice, and the second was the cardiac rehabilitation program I directed.

In my patient practice I began to see small miracles occurring. There was Virginia, battling a life-threatening arrhythmia after a heart attack, who always walked into my office for her monthly follow-up with her face beaming, ready to tell me of the latest blooms in her gardens. All spring and summer she tended her precious flowers, and in the fall and winter she planted bulbs or planned for the next year's growing season. Was it the medicine I gave her that controlled her heart rhythm or was it her love of beauty and her eternal joy and optimism to greet the spring?

Then there was Galen, who came to me after three serious heart attacks had left his heart so damaged that it pumped with only 15 percent of the efficiency and power of a normal heart. I knew the statistics all too well: Half the people with this much damage to the heart die within a year. Of course, I didn't share this information with Galen. Patients are not statistics, and the absolute last thing a doctor should do is take away a patient's hope. So I talked with Galen about the things he *could* do rather than the things he *couldn't*. He and his wife bought a stationary cycle; he started a walking program. He resumed his former hobby of light carpentry work. At first he did these activities only several times a week and often for just a few minutes before he became too short of breath to continue. Later he worked up to half an hour a day *every* day on his exercise program. A deeply religious man, Galen remained active in the church. He and his wife did everything together, and she watched his medicine and diet like a hawk. Last year—twelve years after I started caring for him—Galen finally succumbed to his heart disease.

How did Galen beat the odds? Was it luck or the medicines I prescribed for him? Or was it his faith in God and his determination to live life fully, optimistically, and with courage?

Or there was Walt, crippled by angina. After an angioplasty he started a walking program, shed fifteen pounds, and started to live "my life over for the first time." When Walt first came to me, he was plagued by anxiety. As a young man in his forties with a life-threatening condition he was filled with fear of the future and deep regret for the habits that he believed had contributed to his problems. In short, he blamed himself for his condition.

At my urging Walt entered a mindfulness meditation program. At first he didn't like it. He thought it was so "weird" and "passive," and it made him nervous. Slowly he began to come around, and within six months he was meditating on his own, often in conjunction with his walking program. Two years later he was back to teaching and coaching high school football—the two great loves of his life. He still took medicines, but the dosages were dramatically reduced, and his angina was a thing of the past.

How did Walt succeed? Was it just by chance or did his determination to live life fully and in the present make the difference?

What had started as a whisper soon began to shout to me. Over and over again I began to see that the individuals who beat the odds were the ones who got involved, who believed in themselves, who cultivated optimism and hope, who paid attention to their daily habits. I came to believe in miracles.

Don't get me wrong. I still believe that medicine has an important role to play in helping preserve health and cure disease. I continue to edit a leading intensive care textbook and have seen high tech medicine actually rescue people from the jaws of death. But my patient practice has also helped me understand the power of the human spirit and that good health is a partnership between doctor and patient with the patient playing the deciding role.

My cardiac rehabilitation program furthered this education. Here I had the opportunity to see and study hundreds of patients and observe the positive effects of exercise, nutrition, and stress reduction. This experience in cardiac rehabilitation convinced me that these topics were worthy of study and led me to establish the Center for Clinical and Lifestyle Research.

Over the past ten years the center's research teams have performed dozens of studies looking at how daily habits impact on long-term health. As our reputation has grown, so have the number of people who want to have more control over their lives—to feel healthier, happier, more alive.

What began as a trickle of miracles in my clinical practice has grown to a mighty torrent in the laboratory. We developed a walking test based on the data of four hundred people (a huge study, by the way), and more than two million people wrote to us asking for the brochure. We announced a healthy weight loss study, and the next day over four hundred people called trying to participate. We initiated a yearlong mind-body study, and more than two hundred people joined.

We estimate that over the past decade at the Center for Clinical and Lifestyle Research we have studied more than ten thousand people, and our message has reached and touched the lives of millions more. People have come to us for many different reasons: some to improve their fitness; others to lose weight; still others to become stronger or relieve stress. Whatever the specific reason, they come filled with hope and the desire to be healthier and get more out of their lives.

Time and time again people have come to me and expressed surprise at what they have accomplished. Take Cecile, who came to us to lose weight and left feeling that she had reclaimed her life. She went back to college and finished a degree she had been meaning to pursue for twenty years. Or Bob, who joined a walking study and left feeling better than ever in his life. "If I'd only known how good I could feel, I would have started this twenty-five years ago," he said, vowing to continue walking until the day he died. Or Julie, a participant in a stress reduction study who used the technique we taught her to cope with the death of her father and a serious illness of her mother.

What these people and thousands of others have discovered is the power that simple changes can bring to your health and well-being. They've discovered the joy of living fully, consciously, and in the present. They've discovered that simple changes can bring enormous progress.

And so can you.

WHAT DOES IT MEAN TO BE FIT?

Let's go back to that twenty-seven-year-old man who entered Harvard Medical School in 1975. I told you I was a running fanatic, often running forty to fifty miles per week. I thought I had a terrific fitness program, but I was wrong. Sure, my level of cardiovascular endurance was high, but my program was way out of balance.

I was sore all the time. My upper body wasn't strong enough to participate in many of the sports that I loved without my risking significant injury. Since I was burning an enormous number of calories, my weight remained stable despite nutritional habits that could only be charitably described as lousy. As a first-year medical student I felt stressed out much of the time. My running helped somewhat, but it wasn't enough. In short, I wasn't fit.

There was an even bigger problem with my fitness program that I am embarrassed to admit. I viewed people who didn't exercise at the level I did as lazy and unfit. It was this attitude, so prevalent in the 1970s and 1980s, that discouraged so many people from thinking that their own efforts could make a difference in their fitness and their life. Many people came to believe in the misconception that if you weren't training for a marathon or a triathlon or performing high intensity aerobics, you couldn't possibly be fit. Unfortunately a lot of us who were avid exercisers contributed to this mistaken belief. Today we know a lot better.

I like the definition of "fitness" first put forth by the World Health Organization: Fitness is maintaining or developing the capacity to meet the challenges of daily life. Though simple, this definition incorporates the key ideas about fitness. We now know that having the physical health and spiritual well-being to meet these challenges requires fitness in many areas: cardiovascular fitness, muscular strength and endurance, flexibility, functional fitness (balance, mobility, physical activity), mind-body interactions, the ability to manage stress, good nutrition, and weight management. We also now know that these fitness factors are highly modifiable. All it takes are some simple changes. Let's look at how you can put this approach to work in a practical way.

ASKING YOURSELF THE MOST IMPORTANT QUESTION: FIT FOR WHAT?

People often ask me what's the best way to become fit. I always answer this question with another one: "Fit for what?" What are your goals? What are your individual strengths and weaknesses? What areas do you need to work on to reach your goals? The answers to these questions will have profound consequences for how you approach your fitness program. Fail to ask them, and you could doom yourself to the wrong program and failure and disappointment right from the beginning.

The problem with many approaches to fitness programs is that they don't help you answer these questions for your particular physical condition and lifestyle. For example, the person who needs to lose a little weight should approach a fitness program far differently from someone who wants to improve his or her cardiovascular capacity. The person who needs to be stronger to carry out daily activities must approach a fitness program from a very different perspective from that of the person who needs more activity to lower the risk of chronic disease. A vigorous forty-year-old has entirely different fitness needs from a sixty-five-year-old with arthritis in both knees. There are basically as many fitness programs as there are people with different needs.

That's the beauty of what *Fit over Forty* offers you. On the basis of brand-new scientific information, we have designed a program that will enable you to test and evaluate your precise needs. Then, when you know your answers, I'll provide specific fitness programs and show you how to get started, what to expect, and how to proceed. But first, let's look at the science that makes *Fit over Forty* possible.

THE SCIENCE TO HELP YOU FIND YOUR ANSWERS: THE ADVIL FIT OVER FORTY STANDARDS

In my experience, knowing where and how to get started on appropropriate new practices and habits is the biggest hurdle for anyone starting a fitness program. For people over forty this has been a particular problem. While recent research conducted by laboratories around the world has produced important new insights into fitness and its many contributing factors, we in the scientific and medical community could not effectively advise people over forty about many fitness issues because no one had ever established scientifically valid standards for them. What fitness standards existed had been developed largely on college-age individuals with attempts to extrapolate them to older populations. How strong should the average forty-five-year-old man be? What is normal flexibility for the average sixty-five-year-old woman? What is normal cardiovascular endurance for a healthy seventy-year-old man or woman? Astounding as it may seem, we didn't know.

Now with the introduction of the Advil Fit over Forty Standards in this book, that situation has changed. These standards provide, for the first time, a highly accurate but very simple means of evaluating fitness levels in men and women over forty.

How the standards were established

The massive research project that produced the Advil Fit over Forty Standards was conducted at the Center for Clinical and Lifestyle Research in late 1994 and throughout 1995. With grant funding from Whitehall Laboratories, makers of Advil, we performed extensive testing on 349 men and women. We studied cardiovascular fitness, mind-body interactions, muscular strength and endurance, balance, reaction time, flexibility, walk speed, activity level, body fat, nutrition, and stress—all important components of total fitness. From the data developed on each of these parameters we developed standards for each area according to age and sex. On the basis of the laboratory tests used in the study, we also developed a series of simple home tests that any individual can take to determine how he or she compares with others of his or her age and sex.

Needless to say, my colleagues and I are very excited by the possibilities this research opens for helping individuals improve their fitness levels. But we are not alone. The results of this study have also been received with great interest and enthusiasm by the scientific community because such standards have been so needed. In 1995 we presented the scientific background behind the Advil Fit over Forty Standards at a variety of national scientific and medical meetings, including the American College of Sports Medicine, the American Heart Association, and the Gerontological Society of America. Now, in this book, I am presenting these standards in their entirety to the public for the first time.

The importance of the study

At this point you may wonder why one study has created such excitement in the scientific community. After all, a sample of 349 men and women doesn't seem very large. How do we know that standards derived from this database are valid for the total population of men and women over forty?

Good question. Let's look for a moment at where our knowledge comes from. For much of our data on health and fitness issues and how they affect large populations of people, we depend on epidemiological studies. Such studies generally use questionnaires or sometimes interviews to ask a large target population (often thousands) a set of questions designed to gather information about the issue being researched. Some of our best data about risk factors for heart disease or cancer, for instance, come from large epidemiological studies, such as the Framingham Heart Study, Dr. Paffenbarger's College Alumni Studies, which told us much about the importance of physical activity, and the Nurses' Health Study, which has taught us much about the health of women. These studies give us a large overview, but they depend on self-reporting and have other limitations.

To test more specifically for certain factors, whose importance may have been indicated by one of these epidemiological studies, we go into the laboratory to do a detailed study, with proper scientific design and controls, that will produce more precise findings. Conducting this type of laboratory research is so complex, time-consuming, and expensive that many valuable studies report findings based on only ten or twenty subjects. In contrast, the study that resulted in the Advil Fit over Forty Standards was five to six times larger than any previous study of this type. It was also designed so that all elements complied with the definition of a statistically valid sample. We invested more than a year in this huge research project. Now you can reap the benefits because we have standards in ten important areas that help make up total fitness. Let's look a little more at those component parts of total fitness.

What the Advil Fit over Forty Standards measure: the fitness factors

Fitness is not just one quality of life; it's really a unity of many contributing factors that affect our physical and emotional well-being and our ability to meet life's daily challenges. The Advil Fit over Forty Standards include approximately ten factors that scientific research has shown make important contributions to overall health and fitness. These are the aspects you'll be testing and working to improve. I'll be discussing the importance of each factor and giving you specific activity programs to maintain or improve your fitness in it in separate chapters. But a brief overview of how each of these factors contributes to fitness will give you the background you need to take the tests that will establish your Personal Fitness Profile, our next step.

Cardiovascular Fitness

Cardiovascular fitness—a healthy heart and circulatory system—is the primary key to overall well-being because the heart is the body's engine. You can't go without it. Yet heart disease remains the number one killer of men and women in America. By the time a man reaches the age of fifty in the United States he has over a 30 percent chance of having coronary artery disease; by age sixty he has a 20 percent chance of having suffered a heart attack. Over the age of forty a woman is six times as likely to die of heart disease as of breast cancer. Consequently, cardiovascular fitness is the number one modifiable health consideration for individuals over the age of forty.

Muscular Strength and Endurance

Muscular strength and endurance are also key components of health. They contribute to cardiovascular fitness, to functional fitness (the physical ability to carry out a daily routine), and to weight management. As we grow older, strong muscles make it possible not only to perform aerobic exercise, for example, but also to perform such simple tasks as rising from a chair or toilet and climbing the stairs to a second-floor bedroom. Since lean muscle tissue is the body's calorie-burning furnace, preserving lean muscle helps you prevent weight gain. The average inactive person loses half a pound of lean muscle every year. The good news is that muscles have enormous capacity to increase strength—even after you reach age eighty or ninety.

Flexibility

Inactive muscles become weak, stiff muscles. Stiff, inflexible muscles make it hard to get adequate physical or aerobic activity. Inflexible muscles also affect your balance and mobility. As we grow older, inflexibility is one of the greatest contributing factors in falls. Finally, inflexible muscles are prone to injury. Regular stretching preserves flexibility.

Physical Activity

Let me say this as simply and clearly as possible: *An active lifestyle is a healthy lifestyle. Inactivity is hazardous to your health.* A few years ago the Centers for Disease Control in Atlanta surveyed all the available research concerning the impact of activity on health. They concluded that inactive individuals *double* their risk of heart disease compared with active people. To put this in perspective, that means that by choosing to remain inactive, a person accepts the same increased risk of heart disease as if she smoked a pack of cigarettes a day. And the sad truth about our society is that 60 percent of all adults have chosen to remain inactive.

Functional Fitness

A primary goal of fitness should be good health, and part of good health is being able to function at your best every day. This concept is so important that we've even coined a term for it: functional fitness. Among the contributing factors to functional fitness that we can measure are balance, reaction time, and walk speed.

Mind-Body Interrelations and Stress Reduction

Many of us make the mistake of splitting concepts into categories when we should be looking for unifying truths. Mind-body interactions are one of these areas. We aren't simply bodies walking around without ever-vigilant minds. Nor are we simply consciousness devoid of physical reality. Mind and body are forever one, bound inseparably by undeniable connections. Recent research has helped us understand more about these connections and has shown us how to use the links between mind and body to tap into the body's innate capacity to heal both our spirits and our physical beings.

The impact of stress on our lives is one area that involves mind-body connections. Make no mistake about it, stress is hazardous to your health. I see it every day in my practice as a physician, and scientific studies link stress to conditions that range in seriousness from the pesky common cold to life-threatening cancer and heart disease. Stress reduction techniques tap the mind-body interrelations to bring this factor into control.

Nutrition

As the medical editor of the Television Food Network I field hundreds of questions about nutrition and health every year. Nobody can doubt the multiple links between nutrition and health. In fact, the surgeon general has reminded us that seven out of the ten leading causes of death in the United States have a nutrition- or alcohol-related component. Simple modifications in what you eat can make a significant difference in many health risk factors.

Weight Management

Our country is too fat, and it's killing us! In the past decade the incidence of obesity in the United States *grew* a shocking 34 percent. One out of three adults in our country is obese, and by "obese" I mean at least 20 percent over desirable weight. Over 60 percent of the population is at least somewhat overweight. Please understand that as a physician I am not concerned about overweight as a vanity issue. This is a *health* issue. Overweight causes three hundred thousand excess deaths every year in the United States, making it the second leading cause of preventable death. Being just a little overweight can cause health problems. A weight gain of as little as fifteen pounds as an adult significantly increases the risk of heart disease. The good news is that small amounts of weight loss—on the order of ten to fifteen pounds for most people—if maintained, can result in significant reduction in the risk of disease.

PUTTING THE ADVIL FIT OVER FORTY STANDARDS TO WORK FOR YOU

Now it's time ask yourself the next question, How fit am I? The answer lies at the completion of the next step in your Fit over Forty Program, establishing your Personal Fitness Profile by taking the series of ten Fit over Forty Tests in the next chapter. You'll find that they are fun to do as well as very informative. Go to the next chapter, and I'll show you the way across that bridge to the land of the living.

CHAPTER 3

GETTING STARTED: THE FIT OVER FORTY TESTS

DAN

"There's no way that just walking is going to be any sort of challenge!" Dan, a participant in one of our walking studies, was complaining loudly before his first test session. Overweight and fifty-five, he was sure that "just walking" had to be too easy. After the One-Mile Walk Test at the track, he was singing a different tune, something more in the line of the immortal Cole Porter's "Let's Do It."

No matter how simple the Fit over Forty Tests appear on first reading, I think you'll soon agree with Dan that they produce information and results you can use. The ten home tests are not like tests at school. On these tests *everyone* wins and no one loses. You'll find them easy, fun, motivational, and you'll learn a lot about your body, your fitness, and your health. Don't make the mistake of skipping the tests and moving right into the programs in the book. The tests are the best way to get started on the perfect health and fitness program, for your own background, characteristics, and fitness level, and *that's* the way to get started finally on that health and fitness program you've wanted to accomplish for years.

All these tests were developed on individuals over the age of forty. They all are comfortable and safe and can be done in the convenience of your own home—either by yourself or with your spouse or a friend. Some of the tests are "paper and pencil tests"; others require a minimal amount of physical exertion. Most take less than five minutes to take, and none lasts longer than fifteen to twenty minutes. Minimal equipment is required; I'll give you a list in a moment.

As you complete each test, you will record your scores on the Personal Fitness Profile Scorecard at the end of this chapter. When you've finished all the tests, this scorecard will help you compare your results with others of your age and sex. Then in the next chapter you'll learn how to evaluate your strengths and weaknesses and get started on a customized program to improve your health and fitness.

BEFORE YOU START THE TESTS: A FEW PREPARATORY STEPS

You'll enjoy the tests and get the most useful results if you do a little groundwork before you begin. Preparatory steps include planning your test schedule, gathering the equipment you will need, and preparing your Personal Fitness Profile Scorecard. I also suggest that you read the instructions for all the tests straight through before you begin so that you have a good overview of what's involved.

One more thing: While the tests are very easy, and safe and none requires more than moderate physical exertion, it's still a good idea to check with your physician if you have any questions or concerns about your ability to perform them. To avoid injury, you should also remember to warm up properly before each of the active tests; appropriate directions are given with each test.

Step 1: Planning your test schedule

Plan to take the tests over three days and in the order recommended on page 24. This timing and order are designed to help you avoid the fatigue that could affect the accuracy of your results. You may wish to do the tests over three days in a row, perhaps over the weekend, or every other day.

Recommended Test Schedule

Day 1: Fifty-Foot Walk Test
Physical Activity Test
One-Mile Walk Test

Day 2: Balance Test
Flexibility Test
Mind-Body Stress Test

Day 3: Upper Body Strength Test
Lower Body Strength Test
Nutritional Habits
Body Fat

Step 2: Gathering what you will need for the tests

To make your test sessions go smoothly, you need to prepare these items ahead of time.

Location: Most of these tests can be conducted in your home. For the One-Mile Walk Test you will need to use a track or to measure a one-mile route on a flat, level road. You will also need a straight, level fifty-foot area for the Fifty-Foot Walk Test.

Clothing: Comfortable walking shoes.

Loose, comfortable clothing appropriate for the temperature conditions.

Equipment: A stopwatch (for most accurate results). All timed tests except for the Fifty-Foot Walk Test can be performed with a watch that indicates seconds (digital or sweep hand).

5-pound hand weight or dumbbell.

10-pound ankle weight.

You may purchase these weights in a sporting goods outlet (you may choose to use them later in your strength-training program), or you may assemble your own with socks and rocks or sand (instructions accompany the test).

Yardstick.

Masking tape or duct tape.

Dressmaker's flexible tape measure.

Pencil and paper.

Recommended option: a partner to work the stopwatch, help
read the measurements, and cheer you on.

Step 3: Preparing Your Fitness Profile Scorecard

You will find a blank Personal Fitness Profile Scorecard on page 49 at
the end of this chapter. You may use the blank form in the book or
photocopy it. Though you can fill in the average Advil Fit over Forty
Standards for your age and sex as you take the tests, I think you'll find
it most convenient to prepare the scorecard ahead. Of course, you'll be
filling in your results as you complete the tests. Why not fill in the
average data for your age and sex from the Fit over Forty Standards
tables as you read through this chapter. The tables for each test appear
after the instructions for the test.

THE FIT OVER FORTY FITNESS TESTS

Here are the tests. I think you'll find them both enjoyable and
educational. They are presented in the order I recommend you perform
them.

DAY 1: THE FIT OVER FORTY FIFTY-FOOT WALK TEST, PHYSICAL ACTIVITY TEST, ONE-MILE WALK TEST

You can do the Fifty-Foot Walk Test and the One-Mile Walk Test on
the same track or level road. Start with the Fifty-Foot Walk Test, take a
breather with the pencil-and-paper Physical Activity Test, and then do
the One-Mile Walk Test.

⬚TEST⬚ TEST 1: THE FIT OVER FORTY FIFTY-FOOT WALK TEST

Walk speed has significant implications both for a variety of health considerations and such practical matters as your ability to get across the street in the time allotted for a traffic light change. Walking is both fundamentally simple and, from a biomechanical standpoint, tremendously complex. Thus a test of walk speed can help you determine a wide variety of aspects of your functional fitness, varying from balance to problems with your walking gait or even your agility and reaction time.

The test we chose to use for the Advil Fit over Forty Standards was the Fifty-Foot Walk Test. While this test has been used sometimes in the past in patients with arthritis of the knee, it can also supply very important information about mobility for anybody over the age of forty.

Taking the Fit over Forty Fifty-Foot Walk Test

The procedure for taking the Fifty-Foot Walk Test is very simple. You'll need only two things: a stopwatch that is accurate to tenths of a second and a straight line fifty feet long measured on a flat surface. Either time yourself for the test or ask someone to time you (the latter is probably more accurate).

1. Be sure to warm up and stretch before taking the test (follow the instructions for warming-up and stretching in Chapter 11).
2. Start at the beginning of the fifty-foot line you've marked out. On the command "go" start the stopwatch, and walk the fifty feet as fast as possible (without jogging). Stop timing when you cross the fifty-foot mark.
3. Note your time in tenths of seconds, and record this information on your Personal Fitness Profile Scorecard.
4. To determine how you stack up compared with others of your age and sex, compare your results with those on the following table. Use the proper table for your sex and the proper column for your age.

ADVIL FIT OVER FORTY STANDARDS: FIFTY-FOOT WALK TIME

	Fifty-Foot Walk Time (in Seconds)—Females			
	40–49	50–59	60–69	70–79
Above average	<6.7	<7.1	<8.0	<8.2
Average	6.7–7.5	7.1–8.0	8.0–8.6	8.2–9.5
Below average	>7.5	>8.0	>8.6	>9.5

	Fifty-Foot Walk Time (in Seconds)—Males			
	40–49	50–59	60–69	70–79
Above average	<5.7	<6.0	<6.9	<6.9
Average	5.7–6.7	6.0–6.9	6.9–7.8	6.9–8.6
Below average	>6.7	>6.9	>7.8	>8.6

TEST 2: THE FIT OVER FORTY PHYSICAL ACTIVITY TEST

Here's a really easy test. All I'm going to ask you to do is to estimate your average level of physical activity over the past month on the basis of a scale from 0 to 7.

This test of physical activity was developed by my friend Dr. Andrew Jackson for a project he was performing at the National Aeronautics and Space Administration (NASA). We have used it extensively in my laboratory and found that it not only provides a good estimate of physical activity but also correlates reasonably well with cardiovascular fitness levels.

Taking the Physical Activity Test

1. Review the levels of physical activity described in the "Code for Physical Activity" on page 28, and determine which most closely describes your average level of physical activity over the past month. You'll see that the activity levels range from very sedentary (level 0) to very active (level 7).
2. Record your level on your Personal Fitness Profile Scorecard.
3. Now turn to the Advil Fit over Forty Standards table on page 29 to see how your activity level compares with other people of your age and sex who participated in the project.

CODE FOR PHYSICAL ACTIVITY

Use the appropriate number (0–7) that best describes your general activity level for the previous month.

I do not participate regularly in programmed recreation sport or heavy physical activity.

0   I avoid walking or exertion—e.g., always use an elevator, drive whenever possible instead of walking.

1   I walk for pleasure, routinely use stairs, occasionally exercise sufficiently to cause heavy breathing or perspiration.

I participate regularly in recreation or work requiring modest physical activity, such as golf, horseback riding, calisthenics, gymnastics, table tennis, bowling, weight lifting, or yard work.

2   Ten to sixty minutes per week.

3   Over an hour per week.

I participate regularly in heavy physical exercise, such as brisk walking, running or jogging, swimming, cycling, rowing, skipping rope, and running in place, I engage in vigorous aerobic activity exercise, such as tennis, basketball, and handball.

4   I run or briskly walk less than one mile per week or spend less than thirty minutes per week in comparable physical activity.

5   I run or briskly walk one to five miles per week or spend thirty to sixty minutes per week in comparable physical activity.

6   I run or briskly walk five to ten miles per week or spend one to three hours per week in comparable physical activity.

7   I run or briskly walk over ten miles per week or spend over three hours per week in comparable physical activity.

Adapted and used with permission of the authors: R.M. Ross and A.S. Jackson, *Exercise Concepts, Calculations and Computer Applications* (Dubuque: Brown and Benchmark, 1990).

ADVIL FIT OVER FORTY STANDARDS: PHYSICAL ACTIVITY CODES

	Physical Activity Codes—Females			
	40–49	50–59	60–69	70–79
Above average	>6	>5	>5	>5
Average	3–6	3–5	3–5	2–5
Below average	<3	<3	<3	<2

	Physical Activity Codes—Males			
	40–49	50–59	60–69	70–79
Above average	7	>6	>6	>5
Average	5–6	4–6	3–6	3–5
Below average	<5	<4	<3	<3

TEST 3: THE FIT OVER FORTY ONE-MILE WALK TEST

This is a test of cardiovascular endurance. This is also the first walking test of cardiovascular fitness ever developed exclusively for people over forty. To develop the Fit over Forty One-Mile Walk Test, we studied 1,179 individuals—548 men and 631 women—over the age of forty. By studying such a large number of individuals of every fitness level, background, and age between forty and seventy-nine years old, we were able to develop a test that was extremely accurate yet very easy to take. Since the test involves the simple task of walking, it's safe and appropriate for virtually everyone over the age of forty.

Preparing to Take the Fit Over Forty One-Mile Walk Test

You'll want to wear loose, comfortable clothing that will be suitable for brisk walking in the temperature conditions you will encounter for the test. Also wear a digital watch or a watch with a sweep second hand.

You need to find or measure out a mile on a flat surface with no hills, traffic lights, or other impediments. Probably the easiest way to find a measured mile is to visit a local high school or college. It typically has outdoor tracks that are a quarter mile around on the inside lane, so to take the One-Mile Walk Test on such a track, you need to walk four times around. An alternative is to use your car odometer and measure out one mile on a flat, level road.

Taking the Fit over Forty One-Mile Walk Test

1. Warm up and stretch for four to five minutes (see sample stretches in Chapter 11. Particularly stretch the major muscles of the legs). Warm up by walking slowly, and build up the speed until you are walking briskly.
2. Note your start time, and walk the mile as briskly as possible, maintaining a steady pace.
3. At the end of the mile note your time in minutes and seconds on your scorecard.
4. Estimate your relative cardiovascular fitness by comparing your results to the data from the Advil Fit over Forty Standards in the following tables.

ADVIL FIT OVER FORTY STANDARDS: ONE-MILE WALK TEST

Table 1: Females (All times are in minutes and seconds)

	40–49	50–59	60–69	70–79
Excellent	<14:12	<14:42	<15:06	<18:18
Good	14:12–15:06	14:42–15:36	15:06–16:18	18:18–20:00
Average	15:07–16:06	15:37–17:00	16:19–17:30	20:01–21:48
Fair	16:07–17:30	17:01–18:06	17:31–19:12	21:49–24:06
Poor	>17:30	>18:06	>19:12	>24:06

Table 2: Males (All times are in minutes and seconds)

	40–49	50–59	60–69	70–79
Excellent	<12:54	<13:24	<14:06	<15:06
Good	12:54–14:00	13:24–14:24	14:06–15:12	15:06–15:48
Average	14:01–14:42	14:25–15:12	15:13–16:18	15:49–18:48
Fair	14:43–15:30	15:13–16:30	16:19–17:18	18:49–20:18
Poor	>15:30	>16:30	>17:18	>20:18

DAY 2:   **THE FIT OVER FORTY BALANCE TEST, FLEXIBILITY TEST, AND MIND-BODY STRESS REDUCTION TEST**

The tests today can all be done indoors at home and will give you a breather from the brisk walking you did yesterday.

TEST 4: THE FIT OVER FORTY THIRTY-SECOND BALANCE TEST

Good balance is critical to performing the activities of daily life and to avoiding falls. The test we developed for the Advil Fit over Forty Standards involves the ability to maintain your balance for up to thirty seconds while standing on one leg. While a variety of tests have been developed to assess balance, I believe this is the most practical and accurate.

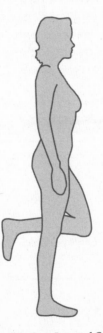

FIGURE 3.1. One-Legged Stance

Taking the Fit over Forty Thirty-Second Balance Test

1. Make sure you have a stopwatch or a watch that indicates seconds. Plan to time yourself or ask someone to time you. Wear loose, comfortable clothing and comfortable, sturdy shoes that do not have slippery soles.
2. Warm up with some light stretches before taking the test (see instructions for general stretching in Chapter 11).
3. The test is very simple. At the command "go" stand on your dominant (stronger) leg with your eyes open and hands resting comfortably at your sides. Maintain this one-legged stance for as long as possible as shown in Figure 3.1. When you lose your balance and your other foot touches down, the test is over.
4. Note the number of seconds that had elapsed when your foot touched down. Alternatively, the test is over if you are able to maintain this stance for thirty seconds.
5. Since the test takes a little practice, you can try it three times and take the best result from the three.
6. Record your best time on your Personal Fitness Profile Scorecard.
7. To determine how you stack up compared with others of your age and sex, compare your results to those in the following table.

ADVIL FIT OVER FORTY STANDARDS: BALANCE

Balance: One Leg/Eyes Open (in Seconds)—Females			
	40–49	50–59	60–69	70–79
Above average	>15.5	>8.7	>4.5	>2.6
Average	7.2–15.5	3.7–8.7	2.5–4.5	1.5–2.6
Below average	<7.2	<3.7	<2.5	<1.5

Balance: One Leg/Eyes Open (in Seconds)—Males			
	40–49	50–59	60–69	70–79
Above average	>14.8	>6.7	>4.0	>3.3
Average	4.1–14.7	3.2–6.7	2.5–4.0	1.8–3.3
Below average	<4.1	<3.2	<2.5	<1.8

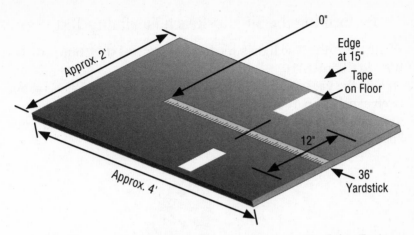

FIGURE 3.2. Yardstick and Masking Tape Setup for Flexibility Testing

⏷TEST⏶ TEST 5: THE FIT OVER FORTY SIT-AND-REACH FLEXIBILITY TEST

The Sit-and-Reach Flexibility Test we used for the Advil Fit over Forty Standards is one frequently used to assess flexibility in younger people. It is very easy to perform, and while it specifically assesses the flexibility of the lower back, hips, and legs, it also provides a reasonable estimate of your overall flexibility.

Optimally the test is given using a simple 15 × 15 × 15-inch boxlike apparatus with a measuring device attached to both the front and the back. Sit in the box as directed, and stretch gently forward as far as possible for a maximum of one second. This apparatus is available in virtually any health club or Y in the United States. Should you have access to one of these facilities, you may use the box apparatus there.

Since many people do not have access to the box apparatus, we've modified the Sit-and-Reach Flexibility Test to make it easier to perform at home. Simply place a yardstick on the floor, and put a piece of masking tape at the fifteen-inch mark, as shown in Figure 3.2.

Performing the Sit-and-Reach Flexibility Test

1. Warm up with some light stretches (see general stretching instructions in Chapter 11).
2. Sit with the yardstick between your legs and with your heels about twelve inches apart and touching the edge of the masking tape, as illustrated in Figure 3.3. Your legs should be straight and your knees flat on the floor.

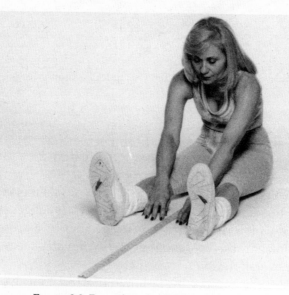

FIGURE 3.3. Procedure for Testing Yourself for Flexibility

3. Reach forward with your hands and arms outstretched for as far as possible, and touch the yardstick, noting the inch marker nearest to where you touch. Perform all movements in a slow, controlled fashion. Avoid rapid or jerking movements, which can lead to muscle pulls.
4. Do the test three times, and record your longest distance on your Personal Fitness Profile Scorecard.
5. Compare your results to the Advil Fit over Forty Standards by using the table opposite.

ADVIL FIT OVER FORTY STANDARDS: FLEXIBILITY

	Females—Sit and Reach (in Inches)			
	40–49	50–59	60–69	70–79
Above average	>18.9	>17.3	>16.8	>16.4
Average	14.5–18.9	14.4–17.3	14.1–16.8	12.9–16.4
Below average	<14.5	<14.4	<14.1	<12.9

	Males—Sit and Reach (in Inches)			
	40–49	50–59	60–69	70–79
Above average	>16.0	>15.6	>13.8	>12.0
Average	12.4–16.0	11.8–15.6	10.0–13.8	9.5–12.0
Below average	<12.4	<11.8	<10.0	<9.5

⟨TEST⟩ TEST 6: THE FIT OVER FORTY MIND-BODY STRESS REDUCTION TEST

This Fit over Forty test shows the powerful interactions between mind and body and how you can use them to reduce your stress level. The test consists of two portions: one to assess chronic stress and the other to estimate acute stress and show you a mind-body technique to reduce it. These tests may seem extremely simple, but research has shown that the perception of stress is its best indicator. In other words, if you *think* you're stressed, you are.

Part 1: Chronic stress

1. To estimate chronic stress, answer the following question by circling the response that best applies to you.
   How often do you experience a great deal of stress in your life?

   Seldom   Sometimes   Most of the time

2. Compare your response with those of individuals of your age and sex by referring to the following findings.

ADVIL FIT OVER FORTY STANDARDS: CHRONIC STRESS

We found that chronic stress was experienced by the individuals participating in the Advil Fit over Forty Standards study on a normal distribution bell curve, with about a third of the participants falling into each category. You can judge your results this way:

Above average: You seldom experience a great deal of stress.

Average: You sometimes experience a great deal of stress.

Below average: You experience a great deal of stress most of the time.

Part 2: Acute stress

To assess your acute stress and employ a mind-body technique to reduce it, perform this ten-minute test.

1. Find a quiet room, free of distractions, and sit down in a comfortable chair.
2. Assess your current level of stress by answering the following question:
   How much stress do you feel right now on a scale of 1 to 10? (answer by circling the correct number).

1	2	3	4	5	6	7	8	9	10

Very little   Average   Very much

3. For the next ten minutes, pay attention to your heart rate and breathing, consciously trying to be aware of and slow your heart rate and breathing somewhat more slowly and deeply than usual. If thoughts come into your mind, don't judge them, but simply let them slip away.
4. At the end of this ten-minute session, ask yourself the following question again:
   How much stress do you feel right now on a scale of 1 to 10? (answer by circling the correct number).

1	2	3	4	5	6	7	8	9	10

Very little   Average   Very much

Unless you started with a very low level of stress, most people will drop one or two points on the scale through this simple ten-minute mind-body exercise.

In our research project we found that stress levels were very consistent for both sexes and through all age groups. If you scored at level 5 or 6 before the ten-minute test, you are average. Any score above 6 indicates above average stress levels, and below 5 indicates below average stress levels.

DAY 3: THE FIT OVER FORTY UPPER AND LOWER BODY STRENGTH TESTS, NUTRITIONAL HABITS TEST, BODY FAT TEST

Today you get to start with a workout and then recover with some simple pen-and-paper tests.

TESTS 7 AND 8: THE FIT OVER FORTY UPPER AND LOWER BODY STRENGTH TESTS

One of our top priorities when we established the Advil Fit over Forty Standards was to develop age- and sex-specific tests to help individuals over forty determine how strong they are compared with those of their age and sex. Using the results from our 349 research subjects, we established the first scientifically valid strength tests and standards for men and women between forty and seventy-nine years old. One test was developed for the upper body, and the other for the lower body. The tests are very simple and provide an accurate estimate of both muscular strength and endurance.

The only equipment needed for the tests is a five-pound weight for the upper body test and a ten-pound weight for the lower body test. Perhaps the easiest way to obtain these is to buy a five-pound dumbbell and a ten-pound ankle weight from a local sporting goods outlet or athletic or fitness supply store. Alternatively, you can make these by weighing out on a bathroom scale five pounds of sand or small rocks in one sock for the upper body weight and ten pounds in two socks (five pounds to each sock) for the lower body weight. In the latter case you'll need to tie the two socks together and tape them over your ankle when you take the Lower Body Strength Test.

⟨TEST⟩ TEST 7: THE FIT OVER FORTY UPPER BODY STRENGTH TEST

The Fit over Forty Upper Body Strength Test is very easy to perform. It simply asks you to perform biceps curls holding a five-pound weight, as illustrated in Figures 3.4 and 3.5.

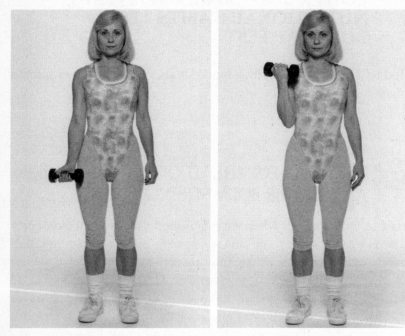

FIGURE 3.4. Biceps Curl: Starting Position

FIGURE 3.5. Biceps Curl: Ending Position

1. Warm up by stretching. (See stretching exercises in Chapter 11.)
2. Lean against a wall, and keep your upper arm stabilized and motionless during the test.
3. Prepare to time yourself for thirty seconds.
4. Begin the biceps curls, and count the number of complete curls you can perform in thirty seconds. To obtain an accurate result, it is important to complete the full movement on each repetition—from the side of your thigh all the way up to your shoulder—as shown in the illustration.
5. Compare your results with the following charts by finding the appropriate chart and columns for your age and sex:

ADVIL FIT OVER FORTY STANDARDS: UPPER BODY STRENGTH

Upper Body Strength and Endurance (Repetitions)—Females			
	40–49	50–59	60–69	70–79
Above average	>27	>25	>22	>21
Average	21–27	20–25	19–22	18–21
Below average	<21	<21	<19	<18
Upper Body Strength and Endurance (Repetitions)—Males			
	40–49	50–59	60–69	70–79
Above average	>34	>33	>31	>28
Average	30–34	29–33	26–31	24–28
Below average	<30	<29	<26	<24

TEST 8: THE FIT OVER FORTY LOWER BODY STRENGTH TEST

The Fit over Forty Lower Body Strength Test follows a similar protocol to that of the Upper Body Strength Test except this time you will be testing your leg muscles. The test asks you to perform leg extensions with a ten-pound weight attached to your ankle, illustrated in Figures 3.6 and 3.7. You need a sturdy table to sit on; the kitchen table or counter usually works well.

1. Warm up with light stretching. (See stretching exercises in Chapter 11.)
2. Sit on the edge of a table or counter with the knees dangling over the edge and the ten-pound weight attached at the ankle on your dominant (stronger) leg.
3. Prepare to time yourself for thirty seconds.
4. Begin the leg extensions, and count the number of completed leg extensions you can perform in thirty seconds. If you are sitting on a counter, avoid bouncing your heel off the drawers or flat surface behind your leg; quick but controlled movement is your goal. To achieve accurate results, it is essential to swing the weighted leg through the full range of motion on each repetition: from vertical to horizontal, as shown in the illustration. Avoid locking the knee in the horizontal position.

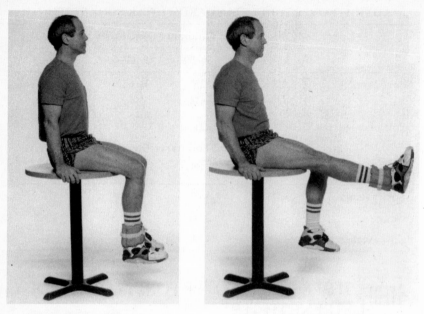

FIGURE 3.6. Leg Extension: FIGURE 3.7. Leg Extension:
    Starting Position   Ending Position

5. Compare your results with the Advil Fit over Forty Standards.

ADVIL FIT OVER FORTY STANDARDS: LOWER BODY STRENGTH

Lower Body Strength and Endurance (Repetitions)—Females			
	40–49	50–59	60–69	70–79
Above average	>27	>27	>25	>25
Average	24–27	23–27	22–25	22–25
Below average	<24	<23	<22	<22

Lower Body Strength and Endurance (Repetitions)—Males			
	40–49	50–59	60–69	70–79
Above average	>31	>30	>29	>28
Average	27–31	27–30	25–29	23–28
Below average	<27	<27	<25	<23

⟨TEST⟩ TEST 9: THE FIT OVER FORTY NUTRITIONAL HABITS TEST

Here's another easy test. Just respond to the five questions about your daily nutritional habits by circling the number that applies to you. After answering the five questions, total the number of points you have scored.

1. How many servings of fruits and vegetables do you eat on a daily basis?

   0   1   2   3   4   5 or more

2. How many eight-ounce glasses of water do you drink on a daily basis?

   0   1   2   3 or more

3. How often do you eat a nutritious breakfast (more than coffee and a doughnut or pastry)?

   0   1   2   3   4
   Never Seldom Sometimes Most of the time Almost always

4. How often do you snack on "junk" foods (for example, chips, pastries, candies, soda)?

   0   1   2   3   4
   Every day Most days Some days Seldom   Never

5. How often do you eat high-fat foods (such as butter or margarine, creamy dressings, hamburger, etc.)?

   0   1   2   3   4
   Every day Most days Some days Seldom   Never

Total up the number of points you have scored for these key practices, and record your number here:

Compare your total with the Index of Sound Nutritional practices in the table below.

ADVIL FIT OVER FORTY STANDARDS: INDEX OF SOUND NUTRITIONAL PRACTICES

Number of Points	Rating
18–20	Excellent
15–17	Good
12–14	Average
9–11	Poor
Below 9	Very poor

⟨TEST⟩ TEST 10: THE FIT OVER FORTY BODY FAT TESTS: BODY MASS INDEX AND WAIST-TO-HIP RATIO

We tested all of our 349 subjects in the Advil Fit over Forty Standards project for obesity. Why do we need special tests for obesity? After all, you might argue that all a person really needs to do is look in the mirror or step on a scale to determine if he or she weighs too much.

Well, yes . . . and no. There are two issues that our tests can help you with beyond the information from the mirror and the scale. One is body fat and the other is where that body fat is distributed. Both percentage of body fat and body fat distribution are associated with health consequences of obesity.

The Fit over Forty Standards Body Fat Tests are Body Mass Index and Waist-to-Hip Ratio. One involves the use of a table, while the other requires a tape measure. So grab a pencil, find the type of cloth tape measure that tailors use (available in a department store if you don't already own one), and let's go!

Part 1: Body Mass Index (BMI)

Body Mass Index is a research tool that is used to estimate a person's body fat. Of course, in a research laboratory we have much more elaborate techniques for making this assessment, such as underwater weighing and the skin fold caliper technique, but as a practical matter BMI provides a reasonably accurate estimate of body fat.

The computation of BMI involves using the fact that height and weight and body surface area are related to one another. The actual formula involves dividing body weight (in kilograms no less) by height squared (in meters). Unless you're a math whiz, you're not going to do this. In fact, I don't know a single physician outside those of us who conduct research in this area who actually computes BMI from the formula. The easiest approach is to pluck the numbers off a table like the one provided on pages 44 and 45.

Using the BMI table is very easy. Just follow this procedure:

1. Find your height in inches in the left-hand column.
2. Run your finger across the page from this height number horizontally until you find your weight in pounds.

3. Look to the top of the column from your weight to determine your BMI.

That's all there is to it. Let me give you an example. Let's say that Sharon is five feet five inches and weighs 164 pounds. Find her height in the left column (5'5" = 65"). Running your finger across to her weight of 164 pounds and then glancing up to the top of the column, you can see that her BMI is between 27 and 28.
1. Now, using this same process, but with your height and weight, determine your BMI.
2. Note this number on your Personal Fitness Profile Scorecard.
3. Compare your results with the following standards. I would give you the results of the BMIs we obtained in the Advil Fit over Forty Standards study, but they weren't very good. The average for both

HEIGHTS (INCHES) AND WEIGHTS (POUNDS) THAT CORRESPOND TO BMIS OF 19 AND 25

Height (inches)	Weight (pounds), BMI=19	Weight (pounds), BMI=25
58	91	119
59	94	124
60	97	127
61	101	132
62	103	136
63	107	141
64	111	146
65	114	150
66	118	156
67	121	159
68	125	165
69	128	169
70	133	175
71	136	179
72	140	185
73	143	189
74	148	195
75	151	199
76	156	205

BODY WEIGHT (IN POUNDS) ACCORDING TO HEIGHT (IN INCHES) AND BODY MASS INDEX

Height	\	\	\	\	\	\	\	Body Mass Index	\	\	\	\	\	\	\	\
	19	20	21	22	23	24	25	26	27	28	29	30	31	32	33	34
								Body Weight								
58	91	95	100	105	110	114	119	124	129	133	138	143	148	152	157	162
59	94	99	104	109	114	119	124	129	134	139	144	149	154	159	164	169
60	97	102	107	112	117	122	127	132	138	143	148	153	158	163	168	173
61	101	106	111	117	122	127	132	138	143	148	154	159	164	169	175	180
62	103	109	114	120	125	130	136	141	147	152	158	163	168	174	179	185
63	107	113	119	124	130	135	141	147	152	158	164	169	175	181	186	192
64	111	117	123	129	135	141	146	152	158	164	170	176	182	187	193	199
65	114	120	126	132	138	144	150	156	162	168	174	180	186	192	198	204
66	118	124	131	137	143	149	156	162	168	174	180	187	193	199	205	212
67	121	127	134	140	147	153	159	166	172	178	185	191	198	204	210	217
68	125	132	139	145	152	158	165	172	178	185	191	198	205	211	218	224
69	128	135	142	149	155	162	169	176	182	189	196	203	209	216	223	230
70	133	140	147	154	161	168	175	182	189	196	203	210	217	224	231	237
71	136	143	150	157	164	171	179	186	193	200	207	214	221	229	236	243
72	140	148	155	162	170	177	185	192	199	207	214	221	229	236	244	251
73	143	151	158	166	174	181	189	196	204	211	219	226	234	241	249	257
74	148	156	164	171	179	187	195	203	210	218	226	234	242	249	257	265
75	151	159	167	175	183	191	199	207	215	223	231	239	247	255	263	271
76	156	164	172	181	189	197	205	214	222	230	238	246	255	263	271	279

From *Weighing the Options* (National Academy of Sciences, 1995). Used with permission.

BODY WEIGHT (IN POUNDS) ACCORDING TO HEIGHT (IN INCHES) AND BODY MASS INDEX (continued)

Height		Body Mass Index														
	35	36	37	38	39	40	41	42	43	44	45	46	47	48	49	50
	Body Weight															
58	167	172	176	181	186	191	195	200	205	210	214	219	224	229	233	238
59	174	179	184	188	193	198	203	208	213	218	223	228	233	238	243	248
60	178	183	188	194	199	204	209	214	219	224	229	234	239	244	250	255
61	185	191	196	201	207	212	217	222	228	233	238	244	249	254	260	265
62	190	196	201	206	212	217	223	228	234	239	245	250	255	261	266	272
63	198	203	209	214	220	226	231	237	243	248	254	260	265	271	277	282
64	205	211	217	223	228	234	240	246	252	258	264	269	275	281	287	293
65	210	216	222	228	234	240	246	252	258	264	270	276	282	288	294	300
66	218	224	230	236	243	249	255	261	268	274	280	286	292	299	305	311
67	223	229	236	242	248	255	261	268	274	280	287	293	299	306	312	319
68	231	238	244	251	257	264	271	277	284	290	297	304	310	317	323	330
69	236	243	250	257	263	270	277	284	290	297	304	311	317	324	331	338
70	244	251	258	265	272	279	286	293	300	307	314	321	328	335	342	349
71	250	257	264	271	279	286	293	300	307	314	321	329	336	343	350	357
72	258	266	273	281	288	295	303	313	317	325	332	340	347	354	362	369
73	264	272	279	287	294	302	309	317	324	332	340	347	355	362	370	377
74	273	281	288	296	304	312	319	327	335	343	351	358	366	374	382	390
75	279	287	294	302	310	318	326	334	342	350	358	366	374	382	390	398
76	287	296	304	312	320	328	337	345	353	361	370	378	386	394	402	411

men and women was above 26.5—higher than I believe is healthy. Rather, I have given you the heights and weights for a BMI of 19 and 25, which is a range of healthy weights. The new national guidelines announced by the U.S. Department of Agriculture recommend that we strive for weights in this range in order to be at our healthy weight.

One final issue related to BMI. People often ask if there are different BMI tables for men and women. The answer is no. The same equation and tables apply to both sexes.

Part 2: Waist-to-Hip Ratio

The second indicator of body fat or obesity that was employed in the Advil Fit over Forty Standards project was Waist-to-Hip Ratio. This measurement provides specific information about where the fat is distributed on the body. This in turn has been shown to relate to the risk of heart disease.

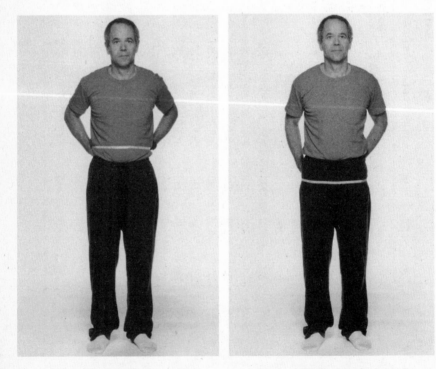

FIGURE 3.8. Waist Measurement   Figure 3.9. Hip Measurement

Of course, there are sexual differences between men and women with regard to the distribution of fat. Men tend to carry more fat in their abdominal regions while women have more genetic propensity to carry extra fat in their hips and thighs. It is excessive amounts of abdominal fat (the so-called apple shape) that is associated with the increased risk of heart disease in both men and women. In contrast, weight distributed at the hips and thighs (the so-called pear shape) does not elevate the risk as much.

Determining your Waist-to-Hip Ratio is a relatively simple matter. It merely requires the use of your cloth measuring tape.

Follow the procedures depicted in Figures 3.8 and 3.9.

1. Measure your waist in inches at the narrowest area above your umbilicus (belly button) as depicted in Figure 3.8. Record the number on your scorecard.
2. Measure your hips in inches at the maximal protrusion of the buttocks as illustrated in Figure 3.9. Record the number on your scorecard.
3. To determine your Waist-to-Hip Ratio, divide your waist measurement (inches) by your hip measurement (inches). Record the number on your scorecard.
4. Compare your ratio with the standards. How do you know the best Waist-to-Hip Ratio for you? Once again, I'd like to say that the results from the Advil Fit over Forty Standards project could help, but the truth is that like many Americans, their ratios were slightly elevated.

Several national studies, however, have provided useful data to gauge your Waist-to-Hip Ratio. Men should aim for a ratio no greater than 1.0, while women should shoot for no greater than 0.8. If you are much above either of these numbers, your risk for various chronic diseases, such as heart disease, diabetes, and hypertension, begins to accelerate rapidly.

It's important to remember that regional fat distribution is largely inherited. However, the amount of fat that is stored can be controlled to a significant degree by effective weight management.

EVALUATING THE RESULTS OF YOUR
FIT OVER FORTY TESTS: CONSIDERING YOUR
PERSONAL FITNESS PROFILE

Congratulations! By now you've completed the ten simple health and fitness home tests developed as part of the Advil Fit over Forty Standards project. You've had a chance to measure your cardiovascular fitness, strength, balance, mobility, body fat, and a whole lot more. I hope you've found the tests both enjoyable and educational.

In the next chapter I'll discuss how you can evaluate your current levels of fitness and use the information and programs in the rest of this book to help you design your own fitness program. Separate chapters are devoted to important aspects of developing a fitter lifestyle and to each area that you measured, such as cardiovascular fitness, stress, strength, or nutrition. In addition, I'll be supplying you with general information on such important topics as mind-body interactions, health and fitness and aging, and how to modify your program if you have a chronic condition, such as diabetes, osteoporosis, cancer, or heart disease.

The poet T. S. Eliot once wrote: "Home is where one starts from." Well, your Personal Fitness Profile Scorecard is where you'll start from. Over the next few weeks, as you work your way through this book and adopt the various programs and practices, you'll be amazed at how far you go. At the end of twelve weeks, once you're well established on your fitness program, I encourage you to take the ten Fit over Forty tests again to chart your progress. A scorecard to record your results from this second round of testing is in the Appendix.

Well, we're ready to go. You've tested yourself, you've packed your bags, and you're ready to start the journey toward better health and fitness. As your guide I've got the maps. Let's head for the next bridge!

FIT OVER FORTY PERSONAL
FITNESS PROFILE SCORECARD

In the column headed "Your Data" record your results on the Fit over Forty tests. In the column headed "Average Data for Your Age and Sex" record the appropriate figures from the Advil Fit over Forty Standards for each test in Chapter 3. Use the final column, "Your Goals," as you plan your fitness program, using the information in Chapter 4.

THE TESTS	YOUR DATA	AVERAGE DATA FOR YOUR AGE AND SEX	YOUR GOALS
1. Fifty-Foot Walk Test for Mobility			
2. Physical Activity Test			
3. One-Mile Walk Test for Cardio-vascular Fitness			
4. Thirty-Second Balance Test			
5. Sit-and-Reach Flexibility Test			
6. Mind-Body Stress Reduction Test			
7. Upper Body Strength Test			
8. Lower Body Strength Test			
9. Nutritional Habits Test			
10. Body Fat Tests: Body Mass Index			
Waist-to-Hip Ratio			

CHAPTER 4

PLANNING YOUR PERSONAL FITNESS PROGRAM

With your Fit over Forty Tests completed, you're ready to ask yourself these important questions that, as I mentioned earlier, will help you plan and get started on a program for total fitness that is right for you:

How fit am I now? What are my individual strengths and weaknesses?

What are my goals for fitness? What component areas of fitness do I need to work on to reach my goals?

Where will I start? What are my priorities?

What's convenient for me? What do I enjoy doing?

As you reflect on these questions and begin evaluating the results revealed by your Personal Fitness Profile Scorecard, remember that the overall goal of Fit over Forty is to help you discover the power that is within you to live fully and healthfully. This new vision of fitness as more than "exercise" or "diet" gives you a chance to take charge of your lifestyle. It also requires that you take time to evaluate, reflect, and plan so that the simple changes in daily habits and the fitness programs that you select are right for you. I know you're eager to get going, but taking a day or two to work through this chapter on planning will save you time and frustration. In my experience, people who have trouble starting or staying with fitness programs don't falter on cosmic or complicated issues. Rather they fail because they don't take the time to ask themselves simple, commonsense questions or take the rather minor steps to prepare themselves, their equipment, and their routine. Don't let this happen to you. A little attention to detail can make all the difference in the world.

In this chapter I'm going to help you do three things: (1) evaluate your Personal Fitness Profile so that you can see where you need work, (2) set fitness goals that are right for you, and (3) plan your personal comprehensive fitness program with the assistance of some specific recommendations and tips.

HOW FIT ARE YOU NOW?: EVALUATING YOUR FITNESS PROFILE

Let's start by taking a look at your Personal Fitness Profile Scorecard. Your results on these tests measuring ten important components of overall health and fitness can give you a good picture of your general fitness for a person of your age and sex, and individual test results can reveal particular areas that need improvement. So get a pencil and paper to note your judgments as you answer these questions:

1. First, look over your test results as a whole. For your age and sex, do most of your scores fall into one category—i.e., below average, average, or above average?—or are they evenly mixed?
2. Next, evaluate your scores in each area. Are you below average, average, or above average? At the top, middle, or bottom of your category?

    How is your cardiovascular fitness?
      (One-Mile Walk)

    How physically active are you?

    How strong are you?

      Upper body strength

      Lower body strength

How flexible are you?

How functionally fit are you?

   Mobility (Fifty-Foot Walk)

   Balance

How stressed are you feeling?

Where is your nutrition profile?

Do you need to lose weight?

3. As you look at your answers to the questions in the previous step, what areas do you need most to work on? Note the area that seems to need the most work first and then the second and so on. Do you notice any correlations between areas? For example, in the Advil Fit over Forty Standards study we found that being physically active correlated with better cardiovascular fitness and the reverse. Similarly, mobility as measured by the Fifty-Foot Walk Test was strongly related to cardiovascular fitness and strength. You will probably find similar connections in your results.
4. Take a moment to think about what your answers to these questions say to you. What do they make you want to accomplish?

SETTING YOUR GOALS

Now that you know how fit you are, it's time to set some achievable goals for the future. Some of your goals may be very specific—for example, "I want to improve my cardiovascular fitness from below average to at least average," "to build my upper body strength," or "to increase my physical activity level from 2 to 6 or 7." Other goals will be more general—for instance, "I want to have more feeling of control over my health," "to enjoy rather than dread my exercise program," "to have more energy," or "to feel a sense of accomplishment." Whether specific or general, your goals should reflect what is important to you and should give you a way to measure your progress.

I can't tell you what your goals should be—that's your job—but I can give you some important tips to help you set really useful goals:

1. Set realistic, doable goals. If you are like most individuals, your Personal Fitness Profile has indicated that you need to work on

improving your fitness levels in several component areas, not just one. As you consider what you want to achieve, set your end goal as high as you like, but set realistic, doable intermediate goals to help you reach that glorious finale. Setting unrealistic goals with impossibly short time frames is an excellent recipe for failure.

2. Plan to take your time, and emphasize the fun. After all, you are trying to make changes that will last a lifetime. So plan to tackle one goal or related group of goals at a time, adding activities to achieve a second goal as you get comfortable with the activities you've undertaken to reach the first. Trying to do too much at once and pushing yourself to the point of tedium or burnout won't work. Remember, if you're not enjoying what you're doing, then it's not really helping you achieve the larger goal of living more fully.

3. Remember that achieving fitness is a progressive continuum. Achieving fitness doesn't mean that everyone reaches one perfect state of being, but that different individuals achieve different benefits. For example, if you are among the truly sedentary and you begin, let's say, to add more physical activity to each day and start the Fit over Forty Walking Program, you will see and feel measurable, even dramatic improvement in several of your fitness levels (and health risk factors) in just a few weeks. On the other hand, if you already have achieved average levels of fitness in most areas but would like, for instance, to become stronger and reach optimal (rather than average) cardiovascular fitness, then your gains won't be as dramatic or quick but they will be just as significant for your health and well-being. Aim to make progress along the fitness continuum toward your ultimate goals.

4. Build on your accomplishments. This tip is closely related to recognizing that achieving fitness is a continuum of benefits. When you have achieved healthy levels, set new goals to go for healthier levels and even optimal levels of fitness and well-being.

5. Never lose sight of the ultimate goal: living more fully and happily than you ever have. He or she who dies with the most toys does *not* win. *Fit over Forty* is about achieving peace with your body and your lifestyle—the real victory—not about beating yourself up to win some imaginary competition with yourself or your friends and colleagues.

6. Write your goals down, and post them where you'll see them every day. This is an excellent way of motivating yourself and keeping

your eye on the ball. It's also a great way of charting your continued progress. You may also wish to use the column headed "Your Goals" on your Personal Fitness Profile Scorecard to note specific goals for each fitness area: what you'd like to have achieved (and realistically think you can achieve) when you've finished your first twelve-week Fit over Forty Program and retest and replan.

With these tips in mind, why don't you take a moment to review your Personal Fitness Profile evaluation and jot down some initial goals for what you'd like to accomplish in your fitness program? You may modify this list as you work your way through the planning section, but it will give you a good starting place.

PLANNING YOUR PERSONAL FIT OVER FORTY PROGRAM

With your goals identified, you're ready to design your personal Fit over Forty Program. As a first step, we're going to review the specific information and fitness activity programs that *Fit over Forty* provides. Then we'll look at pointers for creating a plan using these activities that fits your goals. Finally, I'll share a sample Fit over Forty program that you may use as a planning model.

ALL YOU NEED TO KNOW: THE FIT OVER FORTY PROGRAMS

Each of the remaining chapters of *Fit over Forty* presents either a discussion of an important aspect of total fitness or details of specific activity programs for working on each of the component areas of fitness that you tested. Let's take a brief look at these "building blocks" for your program.

Toward a fitter lifestyle

In the next section of the book—three chapters grouped under the title "Toward a Fitter Lifestyle"—we'll look at three concepts that lay the foundation for achieving your overall goals of physical and spiritual well-being: increasing physical activity, drawing on the power of mind-body interrelationships, and achieving functional fitness (the key to living fully for a lifetime). These concepts are so fundamental and important to planning your program that I recommend that you stop and read them before you complete designing your plan. It's also okay to read them after you've worked through this chapter if you prefer.

Fit over Forty Fitness Programs

In the third section of the book we get down to some nitty-gritty details. Each of these chapters presents specific activity programs to build fitness in one of the component areas of fitness that you tested using the Fit over Forty Tests. These programs were designed specifically for persons over forty and have been tested extensively. We know they work.

Knowing that many of you are poised to push the go button, I've written each of these chapters so that you can use them independently after you've designed your overall program and decided with which specific activity you will start. But if you are the type who likes to read *all* the directions before you start a project, you may prefer to read straight through the chapters to get a good overview. Either approach works.

Here's what you'll find:

Chapter 8, "Walking (and Other Activities) for Cardiovascular Fitness," presents a twelve-week walking program, customized for your age, sex, and fitness level. I recommend this program as the foundation program for any fitness program because walking is accessible to almost everyone, it's enjoyable, it's adaptable to every fitness level, and in addition to promoting cardiovascular fitness, it contributes to many other fitness factors, such as weight management, lower body strength, mobility, balance, and stress reduction. This chapter also offers tips on aerobic programs that you can use for variety or instead of walking. These include jogging, cycling, stair stepping, swimming, rowing, aerobic dance, step aerobics, cross-country skiing, and in-line skating.

Chapter 9, "Stress Reduction: Finding Inner Peace," discusses the various causes of stress and presents principles of stress reduction and a simple but highly effective program to reduce stress that takes just ten minutes a day.

Chapter 10, "Getting Stronger: Programs to Build Muscular Fitness," discusses the importance of strength and endurance to your health and functional fitness and gives you two different strength programs to choose from: a calisthenics program you can do at home and a machine or barbell program that requires the specialized facilities of a health club or Y.

Chapter 11, "Flexibility: Staying Loose," demonstrates how important flexibility is to comprehensive fitness and offers stretching exercises for general flexibility and for use with such specific activities as walking and jogging or strength training.

Chapter 12, "Eating Right: Principles of Sound Nutrition," outlines the basics you need to know to put the principles of good nutrition to work for you wherever you eat—at home or away.

Chapter 13, "Healthy Weight Management," will help you adopt an approach to food and eating that will help you lose weight and incorporate new dietary habits and practices that will make keeping the weight off simple.

Fit over Forty no matter what

No matter how successful you are at making healthful habits and activity routines a part of normal life, two events will intrude: (1) you will have a birthday every year, and (2) you will hit some bumps in the road. In the final section of the book I deal with these fundamental realities. Chapter 14 offers some tips for staying fit as you head toward and pass your sixty-fifth birthday, and Chapter 15 will help you maintain fitness while coping with such special health considerations as heart disease, cancer, diabetes, pregnancy, and arthritis. If these situations already apply to you, read the chapters while you are planning. If not, find time to read them later on and rejoice in the good news. "Be prepared" is an excellent motto for all of us, not just Boy Scouts.

POINTERS FOR PLANNING A PROGRAM THAT'S RIGHT FOR YOU

Well, you're finally ready to plan. As you think about possible activity programs and sketch out a schedule (dipping into the chapters ahead as you need to), apply the following steps (which you'll discover parallel your goal-setting steps):

Before you leap, ask yourself these two questions: What do I like to do? and What would be convenient to do? More people fail at starting activity programs because they choose activities that they dislike or that they can't fit conveniently into their daily lives than for any other reason. If you hate riding a stationary bike, for instance, don't choose indoor cycling as your primary cardiovascular fitness activity even if you already have a perfectly good bike rusting in the basement. If you don't have easy access to a pool, choosing to swim doesn't make a lot of sense.

Some other factors to consider when choosing your activity programs include whether you like to work out alone or need the company of others (a partner or a group), whether you find a quiet walk or jog most calming after a stressful day or need to "beat up on" a bike or rowing machine to release tension, or whether you like to be mostly indoors or outdoors. Try to think of any other factors that would have bearing on your enjoyment and convenience as you design a doable program.

Start with the fitness activities that will yield the most benefits for you and will address the issues that are most important to you. If you're like most people, your Personal Fitness Profile has identified several areas that need work, most commonly cardiovascular fitness, losing weight, and building strength and endurance. In such cases I recommend kicking off your fitness program by adding more physical activity to your daily routine (see Chapter 5) and beginning the Fit over Forty Walking Program because as I noted a few pages back, these basic activities improve a lot of fitness factors at once and build a great foundation for an expanded program.

Add activities to your program as you progress. For example, if a major goal is losing weight, plan to begin the Fit over Forty Eating Plan for Weight Management after you get settled into and are comfortable with the walking program. If building strength and endurance is more important, work on those goals next.

Don't rush yourself; set realistic time goals. A sign over one printer's service desk reads: Orders you want delivered yesterday must be in by noon tomorrow. The hurry-up attitude prevalent today can sabotage your fitness program if you let it. Real progress takes time; you can't rush biology no matter what the claims of popular fitness schemes and weight loss programs that promise spectacular overnight gains but capture only the popular imagination and pocketbook. It's a new outlook on life you seek. Give yourself the time it takes to get it right.

Evaluate your progress, and set new goals from time to time. Of course, positive results keep us all going. So I recommend that after you've followed your Fit over Forty Program for twelve weeks, you take the
Fit over Forty Tests again and check your progress. Twelve weeks
give you a chance to make some real progress. Use your new test
results to evaluate your progress and fine-tune your goals and fitness program.

One final note: I'm big on record keeping. Every committed fitness enthusiast I've ever met keeps track, at least in a general sense,
of his or her fitness program goals, accomplishments, and results.
The level of detail you record is, of course, up to you and will
reflect your personal style. Some of my patients keep detailed daily
logs; other are more casual. Janet, a patient of mine who has maintained a daily fitness program for ten years, gives herself a shiny
silver star on the calendar next to her desk for every day that she
walks. "I like looking at the calendar every day, particularly toward
the end of the month," she exclaims. "It reminds me how far I've
come and makes me feel proud of myself."

A SAMPLE FIT OVER FORTY PROGRAM

Here, as a final guide map for your planning process, is a sample Fit
over Forty Program that incorporates all the steps and pointers I've
given you. It's based on the recommended twelve-week initial
schedule.

Week 1:   1. Take the Fit over Forty Tests.
            2. Evaluate your Personal Fitness Profile based on
                test results.
            3. Think about your goals as you read Chapters 5 to
                7, "Toward a Fitter Lifestyle."
            4. Finalize your goals, and design your personal pro-
                gram.
            5. Write down and post your goals.
            6. Start and maintain a personal fitness record.

For the purpose of a more vivid example, let's say that you, like 60
percent of Americans, have led a sedentary life and your Fit over Forty
Tests show the following results for a person of your age and sex:

Cardiovascular fitness—fair (below average)

Physical activity—2 (below average)

Strength, upper body—below average, lower body—average

Flexibility—below average

Mobility—average

Balance—average

Nutrition—borderline of poor to average

Weight—BMI indicates you are about twenty-five pounds overweight

Stress—low average

After evaluating these results, you decide that you need to design a pretty comprehensive program to work on all areas. Your primary goals, however, are improving your cardiovascular fitness and physical activity levels and losing weight. You'd also like to improve your flexibility and upper body strength. A little attention to stress reduction is probably also in order. With these goals in mind, you design the following program for yourself. As your guide I give it the seal of approval. And you begin work in Week Two.

Week 2: 1. Try to accumulate thirty minutes of physical activity every day.
2. Begin the Fit over Forty Walking Program.
3. As part of the walking program, use stretches from the Flexibility Program for warm-up and cooldown in Chapter 11.

Week 3: 1. Continue physical activity and walking program.
2. Study the chapter on good nutrition, and plan to make about two changes each week in regular eating habits (i.e., eat a serving of fruit beyond breakfast juice each day; drink water rather than a soft drink for lunch, etc.)
3. Read Chapter 13 on healthy weight management, and plan your weight management eating program.
4. Add stretches from the Flexibility Program in Chapter 11.

Week 4: 1. Continue previous programs and activities.
             2. Begin Weight Management Eating Program.

Week 5: 1. Continue previous programs and activities.
             2. If physical activity and walking programs haven't alleviated the mild stress you've been experiencing, try the Fit over Forty Stress Management Program

Week 6: 1. Continue previous programs and activities.
             2. Begin the Strength Training Program using the home program with weights.

Weeks 7–12: Continue all programs and activities.

Week 12: 1. Retake the Fit over Forty Tests.
             2. Evaluate your new Personal Fitness Profile.
             3. Adjust your goals and program to achieve even more progress.

DRAWING YOUR OWN MAP

With these guides, you're now ready to plot your own map to living more fully and healthfully. If you haven't done so as you read through the chapter, get that pencil and paper and start designing. You'll find that Thoreau was right: Affecting the quality of the day, today and all the days to come, *is* the highest art—and the greatest reward.

TOWARD A
FITTER LIFESTYLE

CHAPTER 5

PHYSICAL ACTIVITY: THE MODERN MAGIC BULLET

HARRY

Let me tell you about Harry.

I almost said, "I'm just wild about Harry's lifestyle!" but that part of the story comes later. I first met Harry ten years ago when his family physician referred him to me as a cardiologist. Harry was experiencing dizziness and chest pain, common complaints but often frustratingly difficult to figure out.

My curiosity was piqued when Harry began to tell me his story. Now fifty-six, Harry had started in the construction business as a carpenter after serving in the army during the Korean War and had expanded into general contracting. Over the years his business had grown steadily to the point that he now supervised two work crews of four to six men each.

Initially Harry's work had been quite vigorous since he was the lead carpenter as well as the boss. But as the business grew, he spent progressively more time in administration and supervision and less time driving nails and sawing lumber. He still came to work in overalls and made it a point to visit each work site every day, often pausing to lend a hand with applying wallboard or with framing. It was during these work site visits that he began to notice a mild and occasional dizziness, particularly after carrying lumber or wallboard up a flight of stairs or when holding heavy material or hammering above his head. He chalked it up to "getting older" and "being out of shape." But gradually over two years the dizziness had become more frequent and severe until it now occurred almost every time he exerted himself. Most worrisome to Harry (and to me) was that during the past month chest pain had begun to accompany the dizziness.

Most of Harry's physical examination and initial laboratory work was normal for a fifty-six-year-old man who at 220 pounds was 30 pounds too heavy for his six-foot-one-inch frame. But his cardiac exam was striking. When I felt the chest wall over his heart, I could feel a firm, sustained pressing of the heart on the chest wall every time it contracted. When I listened all over the heart and major neck arteries, I could detect a loud, chugging murmur with each contraction of the heart. An EKG showed evidence of thickening of the heart muscle of the left ventricle, the main pumping chamber of the heart.

I shared with Harry the good news and bad news of my findings. The good news was that I could explain his symptoms. He had classic aortic stenosis—narrowing of the valve that separates the heart from the aorta, the major artery into which it pumps. The narrowing caused the heart muscle both to work extra hard to pump blood into the body and to thicken to compensate for the extra work. The narrowed valve also reduced blood flow to the brain during exertion and caused the dizziness. The chest pain could be coming from the increased demands of his thickened heart muscle, although narrowing of one or more of the arteries supplying his heart might also be contributing.

So the good news was that we had a likely diagnosis. The bad news was that as further testing confirmed, open heart surgery would be required to resolve the problem. A week later Harry underwent the surgery to replace his narrowed aortic valve with a prosthetic one and supply a bypass graft to his one narrowed coronary artery.

This is where the story gets interesting. During and after his surgery Harry, his wife, Monica, and I had numerous, lengthy discussions about their lifestyle. Over the years Harry and Monica had slowly drifted into the inactive lifestyle that plagues over half of American adults. In the early years the physical nature of his carpentry work made Harry so tired that he simply wanted to have supper, watch some television, and go to bed. Later, as business responsibilities increased, one form of fatigue replaced another, and he still went home exhausted. With three small children, Monica also had her hands full and was only too happy to watch TV after supper. Without thinking about it, they had become sedentary. While inactivity did not contribute to Harry's aortic stenosis (almost certainly he had been born with an abnormal heart valve, as 50 percent of adults with this condition are), it certainly contributed to the other multiple strains on his heart: the expanding tire of fat around his belly, his coronary artery disease, and his weak and inefficient muscles. Facing this quadruple whammy of problems, Harry was like a jet liner flying over the ocean with four engines on fire.

As you can imagine, this health crisis and the open heart surgery got Harry's and Monica's attention, but more important, they gave the couple another chance. As we talked together, Harry and Monica realized that while advanced medical techniques could fix Harry's defective heart valve and blocked artery, they would have to take charge of putting out the other three fires. They realized that if Harry did not become more active, his coronary artery disease would probably progress and he'd eventually face more open heart surgery. He was determined to avoid that, and she was determined to help him avoid that consequence. Monica also realized that unless she made some changes, she was headed down the same path that Harry had already traveled. So they vowed to make two changes: to modify their diet to include lower fat, cholesterol, and calories and, most important, to stop sitting around and to start becoming active. That's when I became wild about Harry's lifestyle. In addition to a regular walking program, Harry and Monica joined a square dance group and, most important, increased their activities around home. They planted and tended the large flower garden that they had always dreamed about. Harry went back to a hobby of wood sculpture, and they planned active vacations with their children.

With these changes Harry lost the extra weight he was carrying around, grew stronger and more energetic, and controlled the progression of his coronary artery disease. With an active lifestyle, he put out the three fires threatening him. Some years later during a routine office visit, Harry said to me, "I feel like I lost a heart valve and found my life. I feel younger, happier, and more alive than ever before." Harry and Monica reclaimed their life through the magic of active living. And so can you.

LET'S GET PHYSICAL

Let me emphasize this point again. An active lifestyle is a healthy lifestyle. Inactivity is hazardous to your health.

Physical activity is the closest thing to a magic bullet we have in modern medicine, yet far too few of us are taking the simple daily steps that would result in vast improvements to our physical and spiritual health. Let me give you an example. A few years ago the Centers for Disease Control, the scientific group whose mission is to safeguard our nation's health, conducted a major statistical analysis of forty-three previously conducted studies of physical activity and health. They compared the risk of heart disease in "active" people and "inactive" people. The results were staggering.

According to the CDC analysis, inactive people *double* their risk of heart disease. Even more distressing was the fact that 60 percent of adults fall into this inactive category by CDC standards. Thus with our inactive lifestyles more than half of the adult population of our country is increasing its risk of heart disease as much as if they smoked a pack of cigarettes a day.

And this is just one area in which inactivity is a killer. In fact, by itself inactivity is the third leading cause of preventable deaths in the United States. When you factor in the contribution that inactivity makes to obesity—the second leading cause of preventable death—you can see that we're talking about a personal and public health issue of unsurpassed importance.

But inactivity doesn't have to be our normal way of life. As Harry and Monica discovered, regular physical activity can become a natural, pleasurable, life-affirming part of our daily lives, and in this chapter I am going to show you how. Whatever the goals and fitness program you have designed (or are in the process of designing) for yourself, you can put the information and tips in this chapter to work for you right away.

"ACCUMULATE" AND "MODERATE": ADOPTING A NEW APPROACH TO PHYSICAL ACTIVITY

Several years ago I was asked to serve on an expert panel convened by the Centers for Disease Control and the American College of Sports Medicine to review the scientific literature linking physical activity to health. After two days of discussion and reviewing hundreds of scientific papers, our group arrived at a simple recommendation that was subsequently published in the *Journal of the American Medical Association*. On the basis of an enormous body of scientific literature, we advised every adult to try to accumulate at least thirty minutes of moderate physical activity on most, if not all, days.

Two words in this recommendation are crucial: "accumulate" and "moderate." By "accumulating" physical activity we meant, just as the word suggests, that you don't need to perform one continuous thirty-minute session of physical activity in a day to receive virtually all its health benefits. Rather, you can accumulate this activity in short bursts throughout the day and receive the same benefits. In other words, fit physical activity into the nooks and crannies that each of us has on a daily basis and still receive the wonderful health benefits. Walk the dog in the morning. Take the stairs at work. Take a mind-clearing ten-minute walk at lunch. Park farther away from the store when shopping (you'll even save the time you usually spend searching for a close-in spot). It's easy to see how quickly the minutes add up if they're fitted into normal daily activities.

By "moderate" we meant an intensity level between light and intense. This means performing more than light or casual activities but by no means activities that feel intense or leave you out of breath. A good example is walking. Brisk or determined walking is a classic "moderate" type of physical activity whereas casual strolling would be considered "light" and race walking would be considered "heavy" or "intense" exertion. The same reasoning can be applied to virtually any activity ranging from housework or yard work to gardening. To get most health benefits, you need to have the sense that you are exerting yourself to some degree, but the key point is that exertion does not have to be intense in order to achieve significant health benefits. Physical activity does not have to be a grim and punishing experience in order to yield benefits. Thankfully, the days of "no pain, no gain" are long gone. (From a strictly scientific standpoint they never were!)

PHYSICAL ACTIVITY AND EXERCISE

Here I want to make one more important distinction, and that's between "physical activity" and "exercise." Of course, there is considerable overlap between the two, but they are not synonymous. "Physical activity" can be defined as any muscular movement that uses energy. Sitting in a chair, for instance, is not physical activity, but getting up out of that chair is. Exercise is, of course, a type of physical activity, but we can define it more narrowly as a planned and structured activity in which we repeat particular bodily movements to achieve or maintain various aspects of fitness. Examples of what we typically think of as exercise range from aerobic dance or step classes to regular swimming, cycling, or jogging programs.

There is also a significant emotional difference between physical activity and exercise. For many people "exercise" conjures up negative associations of physical education classes in school that may have been embarrassing, exhausting, or at the very least uncomfortable. While I firmly believe that exercise doesn't have to be unpleasant (quite the contrary), in this chapter I specifically focus on physical activity in order to emphasize the multiple opportunities each of us has every day to be more active and also because it carries fewer negative connotations.

MORE ABOUT WHAT PHYSICAL ACTIVITY CAN DO FOR YOUR HEALTH

A page or two ago, I noted some of the health dangers that physical inactivity poses. I think you'll find it a great motivator to review some of the specific health benefits increasing physical activity has to offer. While the general knowledge that regular activity promotes good health is widespread, few people realize the depth and strength of this association in tackling such problems as heart disease, cancer, diabetes, obesity, and decline in functional fitness.

Decreasing the risk of heart disease

The linkage between increased physical activity and decreased risk of cardiovascular disease is probably the best documented of all the health-promoting effects of an active lifestyle. In addition to the CDC study I've already quoted, there are several hundred other studies, most of them published in the last decade, that conclude that active people have a much lower risk of heart disease than inactive people. Perhaps the largest and most famous of these studies are the Framingham Heart Study, which has followed more than five thousand residents of Framingham, Massachusetts, for over forty years; the College Alumni Study, directed by my friend Dr. Ralph Paffenbarger; the Multiple Risk Factor Intervention Trial (MRFIT), which followed men at high risk for heart disease; and several studies of the patients from the Cooper Institute for Aerobics Research, published by Dr. Steven Blair and colleagues. In all these studies even relatively small amounts of moderate physical activity, if carried out consistently, substantially lowered the risk of heart disease.

It is also important to note that many studies of physical activity have also shown that it lowers such risk factors for heart disease as high blood pressure and high cholesterol or triglyceride counts.

Is there any wonder why I loved Harry's new lifestyle?

Decreasing the risk of cancer

There is also strong and rapidly accumulating evidence that regular physical activity decreases the risk of cancer. Much of this evidence, once again, comes from the large studies of Drs. Blair and Paffenbarger that have demonstrated marked decreases in risks of such common cancers as those of the colon and breast for people who are physically active. A recent study from Stanford showed that women who were physically active for periods of two to four hours a week cut their risk of breast cancer by 50 percent.

Preventing diabetes

The effectiveness of physical activity in the treatment of diabetes has been known for many years. However, only recently have we learned that regular physical activity is one of the most effective methods for *preventing* diabetes in the first place. The College Alumni Study not long ago demonstrated that physical activity reduces the likelihood of a person's developing adult onset diabetes by between 24 and 100 percent. Most important, the greatest reduction in risk came to those most susceptible to the disease.

Achieving and maintaining healthy weight

The evidence supporting a critical role for physical activity in diminishing the likelihood of obesity is so overwhelming that there is no longer serious debate on the topic. I believe, as do many other medical authorities, that the startling and disheartening increase in obesity in the United States over the past twenty years has more to do with our inactive lifestyles than our poor eating habits, although both play a role. Let me put it bluntly: Unless you remain physically active, it's virtually impossible to prevent weight gain, particularly after the age of forty.

Increasing functional fitness

Let me tell you a secret: If you're trying to maintain optimal function throughout your life, the single most important thing you can do is remain physically active. Our Advil Fit over Forty Standards project clearly demonstrated that the level of physical activity was related to cardiovascular fitness, strength, balance, walk speed, and reaction time.

Other benefits of physical activity

I've seen it far too often in my practice to doubt its truth: People who are physically active not only lower their risk of chronic disease, but also enhance their functional capacity and, in general, lead happier, fuller, more energetic lives. That's why study after study shows that people who regularly walk, garden, dance, or perform vigorous work around the house are just plain healthier. Physical activity not only brings a host of physical benefits but also enlivens the spirit.

When you factor in the powerful benefits of physical activity on heart disease, cancer, diabetes, and weight control along with other known benefits, such as improved mental health and reduced risk of osteoporosis, it's easy to see why it has been estimated that inactivity results in 250,000 needless deaths a year. Our poor habits are actually killing us. Fortunately there are some simple remedies.

ACTIVITY MADE EASY

Over the past year baseball legend Nolan Ryan and I have been on a two-man mission to get Americans off their couches and up and moving. The initiative, which is part of the Advil Forum on Health Education, is called the Activity Made Easy Program. I am proud to be associated with Nolan in bringing the important message and motivation to get more active to millions of people around our country. Our goal is really very simple: to show people how *easy* it is to become more active.

Why do we need to keep emphasizing how easy activity is?

Because people are erecting false barriers that prevent them from acting on the good-news message of how simple it is to be more active and thereby more healthy. Let me give you an example. We asked Yankelovich Partners to conduct as part of our program a survey of American attitudes toward physical activity. Its astounding finding was that over 50 percent of adults think you need to participate in sessions of at least thirty minutes of continuous physical activity to derive health benefits. In reality, as we've already discussed, the medical and scientific literature strongly supports that the view *accumulated* physical activity is just as beneficial. Another startling finding was that 53 percent of all adults in our survey said that they didn't have *time* to be physically active. Other surveys show that only 20 percent of adults are active on a regular basis although over 90 percent agree that regular physical activity is good for our health. So we know better. We've got to put aside our excuses and false barriers and get busy.

Since you're reading this page, you are planning to bridge the gap between good intentions and action in your life. Let's begin.

HOW TO PUT MORE ACTIVITY INTO YOUR DAY

How did you score on the physical activity test on your Personal Fitness Profile? If you're like most American adults, you found that your average physical activity level puts you in category 0, 1, or 2. That's far too little activity and means that you're accepting an enormous health risk. Even categories 3 through 5 are not enough. I want everyone to live in categories 6 and 7. (If you've forgotten what levels of activity those numbers represent, glance back at page 28.)

Here's the goal: fitting at least thirty minutes of moderate-intensity physical activity into your life on most, if not all, days. That's the level where you'll derive significant health benefits. It's also the level where I know that you'll start to make a noticeable difference in your ability to control your weight, elevate your energy level, and expand the joy in your life. To do that, you're not going to have to turn your life upside down. All you need to do is to incorporate some of the common activities from the following five checklists into each day's routine and then adopt the ten tips that show you how to make these activities a continuing part of your life.

FIVE CHECKLISTS OF PHYSICAL ACTIVITIES

The idea of these lists is simple: to remind you of how many wonderful ways there are to be active.

I've divided the activities into five major categories, each of which has a table of its own: outdoor work, indoor work, leisure activities, recreational sports, and cardiovascular fitness activities. Of course, these lists aren't all-inclusive, but you get the idea: There are hundreds of activities to choose from to live a more active lifestyle. So mix and match according to the season, grab a few minutes here and there to accumulate thirty, and above all, have fun!

Outdoor Work Activities

Repairing the car

Washing and waxing the car

Chopping wood

Stacking firewood

General construction

Gardening

  Digging

  Trimming hedges

  Planting

  Weeding

  Clearing brush

Mowing the lawn (a push mower gives you the most activity)

Painting the house

Raking leaves

Picking up yard litter or trash

Cleaning gutters

Shoveling snow

Sweeping

Window cleaning

Indoor Work Activities

Carpentry

Cleaning

Grocery shopping

Mopping floor

Scrubbing

Painting walls

Plastering walls

Scraping paint from walls/trim

Standing (working as a cashier, retail sales associate, artist, etc.)

Stocking shelves

Sweeping floors

Vacuuming

Clothes care

    Handwashing

    Hanging out clothes to dry

    Folding clothes

    Ironing

Woodworking

Leisure Activities

Archery

Badminton

Billiards or shooting pool

Bowling

Slow canoeing

Croquet

Leisurely bicycling (5.5 mph)

Dancing

    Ballroom

    Rock/disco

    Square or folk

Drill team/marching band

Fishing

Hiking (no load)

Horse grooming

Horseback riding

Horseshoes

Recreational Ping-Pong

Rowing (slow)

Sailing

Scuba diving

Shuffleboard

Skating

Skiing (slow)

Sledding

Snowshoeing

Swimming (slow)

Walking (3 mph)

Water skiing

Recreational Sports

Baseball (not pitching)

Basketball

Boxing

Canoe racing

Cricket

Cycle racing

Fencing

Field hockey

Golf (walking with hand-
     pulled cart for clubs)

Gymnastics

Handball

Horse racing

Ice hockey

Judo

Karate

Mountain climbing

Racquetball

Skiing

Rowing/crew racing

Soccer

Squash

Table tennis

Tennis

Touch football

Volleyball

Activities That Promote Cardiovascular Fitness

Aerobic dance

Bench stepping (step aero-
     bics)

Cycling (stationary [50–60
     rpm] or outdoor [9.4
     mph])

Cross-country skiing
     (machine or actual)

In-line skating

Jumping rope

Running

Stair climbing

Swimming

Walking (3–4+ mph)

TEN TIPS FOR MAKING PHYSICAL ACTIVITY PART OF YOUR LIFE

"Okay, okay," I hear you saying, "so there are lots of ways to be more active, but it's not that easy. What's the secret?"

I don't know that there's any one secret, but let me share some tips I've learned from my own life and from patients who have changed their lives forever and for the better by becoming more physically active. If you're guided by these principles, I guarantee you that you'll accumulate your thirty minutes each day without even noticing it. In fact, I'll go one step further: If you follow these guidelines, you will *effortlessly* accumulate thirty minutes of physical activity each day, and after a few months of doing this, the only things you will notice will be how much more energy you have and how uncomfortable you are on a day when you aren't active.

Tip 1: *Accumulate, accumulate*

This is the key word. You don't need to carve out a half hour slot in order to improve your health through increased physical activity. Just be on the lookout throughout the day for the multiple opportunities that present themselves. For instance, walk, don't ride, to lunch; take the stairs for one or two flights rather than ride the elevator; sort out that stuff in the basement you've been meaning to get to.

Tip 2: *Mix and match*

Don't get stuck in a rut. There are hundreds of alternatives for healthy activities.

Tip 3: *Remember, variety is the spice of life*

Vary activities from day to day and season to season. Try, for example, a healthy walk in the woods in the fall, planting a garden in the spring, cycling or swimming in the summer.

Tip 4: *Specify time and place*

I've always found routines are helpful. If I establish at least one time and place for physical activity each day, the others tend to take care of themselves. How about a daily ten-minute walk at lunch?

Tip 5: *Include family and friends*

Sharing activities with family and friends increases your likelihood of living an active lifestyle. It will also enhance the health of those you love. Harry and Monica taught me the power of family activities and planning active vacations.

Tip 6: *Have fun*

Laughter is good medicine. If your activities aren't fun, you're not going to do them. Choose things you enjoy and look forward to.

Tip 7: *Be prepared*

I never take a trip without packing my walking shoes. Always be on the lookout and ready for unexpected opportunities to get a little activity. It's really a mindset.

Tip 8: *Seize the day*

If you're always looking for ways to be more physically active, suddenly they start appearing. Look for what you can do today, not what you can plan to do on the weekend.

Tip 9: *Prioritize*

A secret for a physically active lifestyle is similar to that in many other aspects of life. Establish priorities. Things intrude on your plans only to the degree that you let them. Make physical activity a priority.

Tip 10: *Reward yourself*

While the increased energy, joy, and health that you will derive are wonderful rewards, it's also important to acknowledge and reward yourself for this positive health decision: Take a "Hollywood" shower; buy a CD you've wanted. You deserve a treat for your commitment to good health.

HOW ACTIVE SHOULD WE BE?: MODERATE VERSUS VIGOROUS

I'd be remiss if I didn't discuss one final issue related to physical activity, and that has to do with how active we should be and how vigorous this activity should be.

Within two months after my colleagues and I had published our recommendation to accumulate thirty minutes of physical activity each

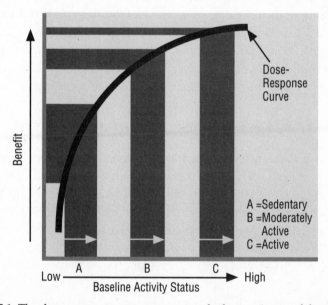

FIGURE 5.1. The dose-response curve represents the best estimate of the relationship between physical activity (dose) and health benefit (response). The lower the baseline physical activity status, the greater will be the health benefit associated with a given increase in physical activity (arrows A, B, and C).

SOURCE: Russell R. Pate, et al., "Physical Activity and Public Health," *Journal of the American Medical Association* 273:5 (1995). Used by permission.

day, another paper was published (also in the *Journal of the American Medical Association*) maintaining that "vigorous" activity was better for your health than "moderate" activity was. The press jumped all over this apparent controversy. I say "apparent" controversy because there is no disagreement among experts when it comes to the health benefits of both moderate and vigorous physical activity.

Let me state the consensus as concisely as I can. If you're currently inactive, *some* activity is clearly better than *none*. If you're already active, *more* activity is clearly better than *some*.

The reason that both these statements are true relates to what in medicine we call the dose-response relationship. The relationship between increased physical activity and health benefits is not linear. Rather, as depicted in the Figure 5.1, it follows a curve.

Thus individuals who are very inactive but start to accumulate even small amounts of activity stand to gain the most. On the other hand, individuals who are already moderately active stand to gain further benefits by becoming even more active. However, they ultimately reach a point of diminishing returns. Most studies support the concept that no additional health benefits accrue to individuals who run or briskly walk more than five miles a day. Beyond these very high levels, these individuals may actually begin harming themselves through injury, fatigue, and burnout associated with overtraining.

TOWARD A MORE ACTIVE LIFESTYLE

In the movie *Rob Roy* one of the hero's sons asks him what "honor" is. Rob Roy responds: "Honor is the gift a man gives himself." If a genie ever springs from that oil lamp I've been so assiduously rubbing all these years and grants me one wish for the health of our nation, I know exactly what I'm going to ask for. "Help everyone become more active," I'll say.

Physical activity is the gift we can all give ourselves.

CHAPTER 6

MIND-BODY INTERACTIONS

PHYLLIS

When I first met Phyllis, she was a mess. She could hardly quit fidgeting as we talked. She was fifty-five years old, and despite having suffered a heart attack four years before, she continued to smoke a pack of cigarettes a day. Phyllis's primary care physician had sent her to me to help clear up a problem that was driving both of them nuts. She was having persistent chest discomfort that occurred both with exertion and at rest and had become so severe it was hindering her performance as a vice-president of a local bank. She was also having trouble sleeping despite increasing doses of Xanax, a powerful and habit-forming tranquilizer.

As I listened to her story, many parts of it didn't hang together. Her chest discomfort could come on at any time, whether she was exerting herself or sitting quietly at her desk. It seemed more common during the day and during the workweek although it occasionally occurred at night and on the weekends. Nitroglycerin tablets under the tongue (a standard and highly effective treatment for angina) had no effect on the pain. The Xanax, while not a perfect solution, seemed to help calm her in the evenings and eventually allowed her to get to sleep.

To try to pinpoint the problem, her doctor had initiated the proper diagnostic workup. Even though he believed that stress and cigarette smoking were contributing to her problem, it was essential to rule out progression of her coronary artery disease. When her exercise treadmill test resulted in equivocal findings (as often occurs with middle-aged women), he referred her to me for further evaluation. A comprehensive battery of tests confirmed our opinion that there had been no further progression of Phyllis's heart disease.

As I shared the good news with Phyllis, I could see the obvious relief in her smile. Together we planned our strategy to deal with what we both could now agree were a series of problems caused by her anxiety and stress. I enrolled her in a smoking cessation program, and most important, I entered her into a wonderful Stress Reduction and Relaxation Program conducted by Dr. Jon Kabat-Zinn, a friend and colleague on the faculty at the University of Massachusetts Medical School. In this highly effective program Dr. Kabat-Zinn teaches patients mindfulness techniques for existing in and fully experiencing the here and now.

Initially Phyllis was somewhat reluctant to try the program. "It seems too passive," she said, "and anyhow, I am the kind of person who believes in mind over matter and solving my own problems." After some gentle urging and some description of success other patients of mine had experienced through the program, she finally agreed to "give it a try."

Three months later, when I saw Phyllis in my clinic, I couldn't believe my eyes. I was looking at a new woman. She had stopped smoking ("piece of cake," she confided) and seemed totally comfortable in her own skin. The nervous fidgeting was gone, and so were the angina and the Xanax. Phyllis had taken the mindfulness meditation taught to her by Dr. Kabat-Zinn and begun to apply it to all sorts of areas of her life. As her mind began to heal, so did her body. "It's hard to even imagine that other person," she exulted. "I feel like I'm finally and fully alive."

MIND-BODY MAGIC

In a sense Phyllis's transformation should not have surprised me. I had seen many other patients experience similar epiphanies when they applied the healing power of their minds to mental and physical problems. Somehow, however, the dramatic and rapid success she achieved helped me focus on what subsequently developed into a major clinical and research issue for me, the healing power of the linkages between mind and body.

Although we have known for many years that multiple and important linkages exist between the mind and body, only recently have we scientists begun to study these relationships seriously and put them into use to help people's lives. Among the many exciting areas of research in medicine, I can't think of a single one with more potential than striving to unlock the secrets of the mind-body relationship to help people turn the power of their minds to the healing process.

My own experience with the power of the mind-body relationship began from my earliest days as a physician. Even as an intern and resident caring for desperately ill patients in a university teaching hospital I seemed to see no clear medical reason for apparently miraculous cures that happened almost daily or for the unexpected disasters that, thankfully, occurred much less frequently. There was George, who walked away from quintuple bypass surgery followed by acute appendicitis, all with a heart operating at a 20 percent level of efficiency. "Don't give away my bed, Doc," he had said with a wink at me when he was wheeled to the operating room for major abdominal surgery less than a week after miraculously surviving five bypass grafts with such a poorly functioning heart. Or take Vicky, who survived heart failure, sepsis, and kidney failure by "never giving up hope." Or Pauline, who survived diabetic coma and shock because "I wanted to see my grandchildren again." After a while I made it a practice to counsel every patient undergoing major surgery or suffering a critical illness not to give up his or her hope and fighting spirit. Often it was the best thing he or she had going for him or her.

In these experiences the power of the mind seemed to have an impact on physical well-being. But I had also noticed that through physical activity and exercise the body seemed to exert a powerful influence on both mental outlook and a sense of spiritual well-being. This interest in mind-body interactions deepened when we began to study the effects of exercise and other lifestyle decisions and practices in my research laboratory. Over and over again research subjects would come to me at the end of the studies on exercise or weight management and proclaim that they felt happier, calmer, more in control, and better about themselves than ever before in their lives.

While I was naturally pleased by this response, at first it perplexed me. After all, the end points of these studies had been improved cardiovascular fitness or lower body weight, *not* improved emotional well-being. Yet the major benefit that most people perceived was in their mood, self-esteem, and mental outlook. It certainly was something intriguing and worth studying, so we did. Over the past five years we have conducted a number of studies that have confirmed amazing links between mind and body and produced powerful techniques that can be applied to elicit mind-body responses.

As I said at the beginning of this book, fitness is not just about taking care of our bodies; it's also about taking care of our spirits. You can't separate the two; our minds and bodies are inextricably linked into a whole. Your attitude and emotional health can have an impact on your physical health, as the examples I shared from my practice show, and being physically active can improve your mental outlook and sense of emotional well-being, as our research has proved. In this chapter I'll tell you about some of these linkages we've found between exercise and emotional well-being and teach you some of the techniques we've developed to enhance the benefits. I'll also share other habits and practices that use the mind-body connection to enhance health and well-being. As you read, think about ways you can use these insights and techniques to help you achieve your goal of a fitter lifestyle.

IN THE ZONE: PHYSICAL ACTIVITY AND THE MIND

Most of us have long had an intuitive sense about mind-body relationships—both negative and positive. How many headaches have you attributed to stress, for example? On the positive side, we've talked about runner's high for many years. And folk wisdom has always said that if you're upset, go for a walk; it will settle you down and make you feel calmer. Now research is confirming those intuitions. When I began to study the positive mind-body relationships in the laboratory, it seemed natural to start with the effects of walking programs because (1) it was walking program participants who were coming to tell me how much happier they were after exercising and (2) walking is an activity available to almost everyone. As an avid runner for years I could also identify with this reaction because I had personally experienced runner's high on many occasions and heard many other runners mention it.

As I thought about it, runner's high seemed like the ultimate expression of a more common mind-body benefit that we could tap into more often through a variety of activities if we could scientifically support the experience that the walkers were reporting. Even if you've never jogged a step, you've probably experienced a feeling similar to runner's high. So what do we mean by runner's high? Though it's been described in many different ways, let me tell you how I experience it. At its deepest, runner's high has to do with a sensation you get once in a blue moon. You're running along, and all of a sudden an afterburner seems to kick in. You feel as if the wind is at your back and as if you could run forever and never tire. You float above the ground. Your mind begins to float as well. A wonderful mellow calm descends upon you. Yet you seem aware of every sight and smell and feeling around you. Everything around you seems to move in slow motion. You feel happy, calm, and free.

This feeling of true runner's high is extremely rare. In all the years that I've been running, I've probably experienced it only four or five times and usually only for brief periods—probably no more than a minute or two. Yet so profound is the feeling that it is something you never forget.

A similar feeling happens upon occasion to many elite athletes. Athletes as diverse as the golf great Jack Nicklaus, basketball legend Larry Bird, and soccer marvel Pelé have described fleeting moments when everything seems to go perfectly, miraculously, exactly as they hoped and dreamed. While their words differ slightly, the concepts all three use to describe the sensation are remarkably similar. There is a sensation of intense calm and total well-being. There is a sensation of both attachment and detachment, of being aware of everything. Everything around them seems to move in slow motion. Athletes have described this wonderful sensation as being in the zone, and they attribute many phenomenal athletic achievements to the rare moments when they ascend to it.

If true runner's high is extremely rare, milder forms are extremely common. In the thousands of runs that I've taken I can't recall a single time when I haven't felt mentally and emotionally better at the end of the run than at the beginning. We know that vigorous activity for someone who is a regular exerciser is one of the very best ways of relieving anxiety and improving mood. Let me tell you a little secret. Even though as a cardiologist I am very well aware that my exercise sessions are good for cardiovascular fitness and, in the long term, lower my risk of heart disease, the driving force that impels me to exercise on a daily basis is the mental benefit. Indeed, surveys show that the major reason two thirds of regular exercisers perform their exercise sessions is that reliable mental lift they get from them. Talk about mind-body connections!

But I am getting ahead of myself. Let's get back to that "walker's high."

PROVING THE EXISTENCE OF A WALKER'S HIGH

When we first proposed a study of a walker's high produced by moderate exercise, there was some skepticism because all studies of runner's high seemed to indicate that vigorous exercise was required to elicit the mind-body interaction. Yet as more and more people from our more gentle walking studies continued to describe similar mental benefits, the stage was set for us to study and attempt to verify walker's high.

Our initial study consisted of forty individuals whom we studied under the following five conditions: fast walking, moderate walking, slow walking, walking at a self-selected pace, and a control condition (no walking session). In each instance the individual came into our laboratory and walked on a treadmill for forty minutes. Before and after the walking session each took a battery of psychological tests to evaluate anxiety and many aspects of his or her mood. We then outfitted our subjects with beepers, and they went back to their normal work environments or daily routines. We paged them every thirty minutes for the next two hours, and they returned to the laboratory to take more psychological tests.

The experimental conditions were carefully chosen to be as neutral as possible. For example, we chose indoor walking to avoid the known benefit of the pleasure that comes from being outdoors. Laboratory members wore white coats and kept interactions with the subjects to a minimum, since we know that certain colors and interactions with others can stimulate psychological responses. We specifically chose the rather long walking period of forty minutes because we didn't want to miss finding a walker's high if it took that long to achieve, although as you will learn later in the chapter, we now have evidence that periods as short as ten minutes are probably effective.

The results of the research were astounding. Speed didn't matter. At any walking speed individuals received immediate and significant mind-body benefits. Anxiety was dramatically reduced, fatigue lessened, vigor increased, and tension decreased. And most important, these mind-body benefits persisted for as long as we continued to monitor our subjects over the next two hours—even after they returned to their work environments.

We had for the first time provided scientific proof for the existence of walker's high.

WHY EXERCISE BENEFITS THE MIND

There are several theories for the underlying links between exercise and the mind, all of which probably contribute to the benefits we experience. Some investigators believe the linkage comes through a class of hormonelike substances called endorphins. These "feel-good" chemicals are thought to be manufactured by the body in a variety of circumstances, such as exercise. They are dumped into the bloodstream and travel to the brain, where they attach to the same receptors thought to be activated by various narcotics. By providing a natural stimulation to these receptors, these chemicals may exert their calming effect.

While the endorphin hypothesis is very attractive as an explanation for the calming and mood-elevating effects of exercise, there are some holes in the theory, and I believe there's more to the mind-body process of exercise than can be explained by one class of chemicals. While these chemicals have been demonstrated in the brains of animals after exercise, the only evidence we have in humans comes from elevated levels of endorphins in blood found in individuals following exercise.

Another explanation for mind-body benefits of exercise comes from the time-out hypothesis. According to this theory, what you're doing when you exercise is taking time away from the stresses and strains of your daily life. Released from these constraints, your mind floats freely and experiences calming and mood-elevating benefits from this pleasant journey. Support for the theory comes from a series of experiments that showed that just relaxing in a recliner resulted in measurable decreases in anxiety. Furthermore, we all know from personal experiences that merely getting away from work or stressful situations will help us put things in perspective. While there is an element of truth in the time-out theory, I think it falls short of explaining the mind-body benefits of exercise. When we've conducted experiments simply getting people away from their work environment and comparing that exercising, the mind-body benefits have been much larger after exercise, more consistent, and much longer-lasting.

A third explanation for the mind-body benefits of exercise comes from the natural body rhythms hypothesis. According to this theory, when you exercise, you move your muscles in a rhythmic fashion and touch on underlying natural bodily rhythms that calm the mind and elevate the mood.

There is certainly some validity to this theory. Use of naturally occurring body rhythms has been an effective technique to help high-level athletes focus on the here and now and relax. Tennis players are often taught to focus on the rhythmic timing of their breathing as a way of relaxing between points. We use the same technique to relax patients undergoing difficult or painful procedures in the cardiac catheterization laboratory. Tibetan monks have used awareness of their rhythmic heartbeats for many centuries as part of their meditative practices; and in the program for stress reduction, described later in this book, we've given a modern twist to this practice to turn it into a highly effective technique for stress reduction.

So what's the bottom line? What really causes the mind-body benefit that reliably occurs with exercise? The truth is we don't really know for sure. It is probably a combination of the three theories I've already discussed plus some other factors yet to be discovered. It is an area of active research in my laboratory and others around the world that will probably greatly expand our knowledge.

In the final analysis, for most of us it doesn't matter *why* both the mind and the body benefit from exercise. What's important is to recognize that physical activity and exercise are wonderful techniques to enhance both mental processes and physical health. It is kind of like getting two for the price of one.

EXPANDING THE MIND-BODY BENEFITS OF EXERCISE

Once we had demonstrated that something as simple as gentle walking could stimulate important mind-body benefits, I was eager to explore the issue further. If something as simple as walking could bring these benefits, what could we do to enhance the process further? Were there techniques that would more reliably evoke the mind-body benefit? How could we make the calming and mood-elevating effects even more profound?

The reason for my excitement was that in the mind-body interaction we had finally found a benefit that occurred *immediately*, not something that required weeks or months for beneficial effects to occur. It seemed the perfect antidote to the problem that many people had with getting discouraged over lack of progress and stopping their exercise programs. But we needed to find ways to help people recognize and enhance the benefits.

Soon I was engaged in an animated series of discussions about this concept and started to incorporate these thoughts into public presentations. After one such presentation my friend Ruth Stricker approached me to follow up the idea. "I like what you're talking about," she said, "and I can help."

Ruth runs a fantastic facility in Minnetonka, Minnesota, called the Marsh: A Center for Balance and Fitness. She has devoted her professional life to exploring the practical applications of the mind-body interface. At her inspiring facility overlooking a lovely wetland she teaches people to find both spiritual and physical harmony through exercise, dance, meditation, and other modalities. Ruth and her husband, Bruce Dayton, agreed, through their foundation, to support the largest mind-body study ever undertaken. It's called the Ruth Stricker Mind-Body Study.

This study, which Ruth helped develop, explored ways of enhancing mind-body interactions. We recruited 161 individuals, men and women, to participate in a yearlong study. The subjects were divided into five different groups, two walking at different intensities, two exercising with an added mental strategy designed to enhance the mind-body interactions, and one serving as controls who were asked not to change any aspect of their lifestyles.

At the end of the study, while all the exercise groups achieved some mind benefits, the two groups that combined exercise with mental strategies (also known as cognitive strategies) had substantially more benefits. These individuals felt more positive and significantly less anxious. They also experienced significant improvement in their life satisfaction and self-esteem.

The two mental strategies chosen were designed both to engage the individuals' minds as part of the exercise process and to pull them firmly into the here and now. One strategy was based on Dr. Herbert Benson's relaxation response. These individuals were given a simple strategy of repeating the words "left" and "right" every time their left or right foot touched down. If other thoughts entered their mind, they were counseled not to judge these thoughts but to let them go and resume their "left, right" mantra.

The other mental strategy involved tai chi exercise, a gentle Chinese movement that contains a meditational form of mental concentration.

The Ruth Stricker Mind-Body Study further convinced me that the mind-body communications we had previously observed with walking were very real and powerful and could be enhanced by some simple mental strategies. Using these findings, I developed a few easy techniques that I now incorporate in my own exercise and teach to people who come to the laboratory to participate in our exercise.

PUTTING MENTAL STRATEGIES TO WORK TO ENHANCE YOUR FITNESS PROGRAM

Here are three simple steps to help you use the mind-body connection to get even more out of your fitness program.

1. *Find a mental strategy that works for you.* While we happened to choose the relaxation response and the mental framework that accompany tai chi, I believe other strategies will also work well. Visualization, mental rehearsal of your exercise routine, meditation, or simply paying attention to your breathing all should work. For example, one of my patients says that during her workout she visualizes herself as a glorious aerobic animal like a cheetah, another sees himself in the most beautiful place he can imagine, and yet others mentally preview their routines and their success. By focusing on their breathing—in and out, in and out (like marching to "left, right, left, right")—still other exercisers pull themselves into the here and now, screening out distractions and stressful thoughts. The point of these strategies is to engage your mind as part of the process and position yourself fully in the present.

2. *Find a specific way of incorporating your mental strategy into your exercise routine.* For most people the best way to accomplish this is to make a conscious effort to start your mental strategy during your warm-up and stretching and then to pick it up again during your cooldown. After a while you'll find that it has inevitably crept into your actual exercise session.

3. *At the end of your exercise session close your eyes for ten to fifteen seconds, and simply experience what you're feeling; take an inventory of your emotions.* This short exercise will help you underscore the immediate mind-body benefits that occur after every exercise session. When I have asked patients in my clinic or research subjects at my laboratory to do this, they invariably report such feelings as "I feel calm" or "I feel happy" or "I feel at peace"—even after their first

exercise sessions. Though it is a very simple thing to do, I have come to think of these ten to fifteen seconds at the end of an exercise session as the most important part of the workout. That little respite reminds us of the multiple links between mind and body and that when we exercise, we bring benefit to both.

But exercise is not the only way you can enhance these wonderful benefits.

STRATEGIES BEYOND EXERCISE FOR DRAWING ON THE BENEFITS OF MIND-BODY RELATIONSHIPS

Research and experience have shown that there are a number of ways beyond exercise that we can use mind-body relationships to enhance our physical and emotional well-being. I encourage you to incorporate these aspects also into your overall program.

Pets, gardens, and dancing

The Irish poet W. B. Yeats once said that the hallmarks of a civilized individual were keeping a domestic pet and maintaining a garden. With apologies to Mr. Yeats, I'd say that's also a pretty good prescription for someone trying to live mindfully and experience the benefits of the mind-body connection.

I'm the proud owner of two large yellow Labrador retrievers and have maintained flower gardens for years. I can't imagine life without either. My dogs, Walker (guess how he got his name!) and Bucky, provide constant companionship on runs and walks and simple friendship, trust, and love. Our outdoor gardens provide fresh flowers six months out of the year, and our indoor plants take over in the fall and winter. Our flowers and flowering plants are constant sources of beauty and wonderful sights, smells, and sounds as well as the home for innumerable butterflies, birds, chipmunks, and squirrels that inhabit our outdoor gardens. Our gardens and pets have brought incomparable joy to my wife and me. And guess what? They're good for our health.

Studies have shown decreases in both blood pressure and heart rate in individuals while they are petting their animals. People with pets are more likely to survive heart attacks than individuals who live alone, and in general, pet owners have longer life expectancies.

Individuals in chronic care facilities have shown dramatic improvements in mental faculties when given the responsibility (and pleasure) of taking care of pets. What makes pet ownership so healthy? I don't think anyone will ever know for sure, but it certainly has something to do with the healing power of love and the mind-body relationships. As a physician I can tell you that my patients with pets invariably do better. I am convinced that pets do more good for us than anything we do for them. Just don't tell my dogs!

What about gardens? The major National Institutes of Health–funded study called the Multiple Risk Factor Intervention Trial (MRFIT) showed that individuals who gardened on a regular basis significantly lowered their risk of heart disease. How could this be? Was it because their cardiovascular fitness level improved? Were they doing "aerobic gardening"? I doubt it. Of course, anyone who does serious gardening knows that there is physical work involved, and it can be quite vigorous. Yet I don't think it's the physical aspects of gardening that make it so healthy. I think it has something to do with the spiritual well-being associated with working the soil, planting the seeds, and watching the fruits (or vegetables or flowers) of your labors grow and prosper. Gardeners are optimists, and optimists live longer. They're also connected to the earth. I remember Leo and Florence, a couple in their seventies for whom I cared for many years. They owned a large farm in western Massachusetts and grew the juiciest, most delicious apples and peaches I ever tasted. Every year they brought me fruit as it was harvested. I think I looked forward to their clinic visits more than they did. Despite their both having severe heart disease, they lived well into their eighties. I'm absolutely convinced that their orchard and their love for the land and each other added ten years to their lives. Perhaps we ought to coin a phrase to describe the health promotion benefits of gardening. How about "mind-body gardening"?

As I have already mentioned, I am one of those people who believe in the immortal words of the cartoon character Snoopy that "To dance is to live!" And there is scientific evidence to back Snoopy and me up. The Multiple Risk Factor Intervention Trial also showed that individuals who regularly danced lowered their risk of heart disease. Now, dancing is terrific for exercise and improving cardiovascular fitness, so that undoubtedly plays a role, but it is also a form of joyful exercise and expression and a powerful way to evoke positive mind-body responses—good for both body and soul.

Getting out of doors

Why is outdoor exercise so pleasant? Why do we feel better on sunny days? Why are some people so depressed during the short days of winter that they actually develop a medical disorder (seasonal affective disorder) that rapidly responds to light?

We all are connected to the environment. In the 1990s we have seen a marked and I believe wonderfully healthy trend back to the outdoor environment. Sales of hiking shoes, mountain bikes, and four-wheel-drive vehicles all have skyrocketed in the past five years—indications that people are spending more time in the outdoors. The likely beneficiary? In my opinion, it is our health. In fact, in my laboratory we've become so interested in this trend that we've coined a term for off-trail outdoor walking. We call it rugged walking, and we have begun the serious study of the multiple health benefits associated with outdoor exercise.

What makes outdoor exercise so beneficial? Nobody knows for certain, but the benefits are so commonly experienced that they're impossible to ignore. Whatever they are, they certainly encompass both mind and body. If I had to guess at the basis of the mind-body benefit of outdoor activity—of course, this is pure speculation—it would have to do with some ancient consciousness that the outdoor environment invokes in all of us. Perhaps it is a little like the line from the haunting song "Colors of the Wind" that Pocahontas sings in the movie *Pocahontas*: "We are all connected to each other, in a circle, in a hoop that never ends." Maybe being outdoors reminds us of the interdependence and connectedness of all living things.

"Reach out and touch someone"

A few years ago AT&T used this catchy slogan to encourage all of us to spend more money with it by making more phone calls. That may have been good for its profits, but the advice was also good for us because it was also promoting a wonderful technique for using mind-body interactions to promote good health! Just ahead of its time, I suppose!

In the last few years a wealth of evidence has accumulated about the health benefits of stable family life and supportive friendships. Men over the age of fifty who are happily married live longer than single men. Is it just the home cooking? It probably is—if you take that term in its broadest sense to include a sense of home, belonging, being loved, and having a close, supportive companion.

Individuals who have survived a heart attack are 30 percent more likely to survive five years if they are involved in stable relationships or living with close friends. Social isolation predicts both mental and physical deterioration and the end of independent living at a younger age for people in their seventies and older than for people who are connected to friends and families. The evidence goes on and on.

What's so healthy about connections to other people? There are lots of theories. Maybe it is stress reduction or lowered blood pressure or just the presence of a caring person to share dreams and frustrations. Maybe there's a link through the immune system. The white blood cells, the main infection fighters and cancer surveillance system in the body, are both more active in socially connected adults than in people who live alone. Whatever the underlying connection, it involves both the mind and the body.

One thing is for certain. We're meant to be social animals. I can often predict a patient's outcome to some degree from the links I observe between him or her and his or her family. Little did AT&T know when it produced its catchy jingle that reaching out to touch someone is one of the healthiest practices around.

The third place

It's been said that every healthy adult has established a solid third place in his or her life, and I believe it is true. We all have our homes and our families as well as the places where we work. In essence, we almost invariably establish the first two places early in life.

So what's the third place? It's the place we go to be with other people who share our interests, hopes, dreams, beliefs, and approach to life. The third place is a kind of spiritual home. It's where we go to satisfy our need for community. For many people the third place always has been the church. For others it may be a health club, a social club, or a volunteer organization. The unifying theme behind active participation in any of these organizations is the sense of community they provide.

Over my years as a physician I've been continuously impressed by the spiritual and health values that people derive from community. Somehow interpersonal relationships, bonding with and caring about others and cultivating spiritual well-being, go hand in hand with physical health and resistance to disease. One patient, Mildred, has always epitomized this for me.

I first started seeing Mildred when she was eighty-two years old. Her previous doctor had retired, and she came to me seeking someone "younger" who could take care of her heart for a long time since she intended to be around for a long time. Mildred had a heart murmur and occasional chest discomfort but otherwise was going strong. She had retired as a schoolteacher from the local school system at the mandatory retirement age of seventy. But rather than slow down, she had used the extra time to devote her enormous energy to the church youth group she led.

For about six months I tried to slow her down. I was concerned about her working with teenagers and having to climb up and down the two flights of stairs at her church. She steadfastly resisted me, saying, "What else is an old woman going to do, sit at home and knit? Anyway, those kids need me."

It finally dawned on me that she was right. Far from being dangerous for her, her church work was what kept Mildred alive. It was what gave meaning and purpose to her life, and that translated into great energy and good health. At eighty-nine she's still going strong with no signs of letting up.

Mildred's story is not unique. In fact, a fascinating body of medical literature has grown up about the health benefits of community ties in general and volunteer work in particular. In one study of over ten thousand individuals in California, membership in a volunteer organization was one of the factors that predicted low mortality. In another, volunteers were shown to have lower risks of a variety of chronic diseases.

Isn't it wonderful to know that doing good for others is a wonderful way of enhancing your personal health and well-being?

MINDFULNESS

In one way or another all the mind-body connections that I have discussed in this chapter have to do with living each day fully and consciously and recognizing the powerful connections between mind and body. Far too many of us suffer from the misconception that mental or spiritual health and physical well-being are separated entities. When we do this, we set up a false dichotomy and don't take advantage of the powerful healing forces within our own bodies.

As a physician and researcher over the past twenty years I have seen and studied too many examples of the powerful links between mind and body to ignore them. Our bodies have an innate wisdom and phenomenal healing power if we only learn to tap into it.

There is no doubt in my mind that the links between body and mind are real and powerful. Each of us simply needs to find our own path to discover them. Whether we choose exercise, gardening, friendships, or volunteer work, each of us has many options and paths toward enhancing these powerful mind-body relationships. The key is to recognize that they are there in the first place. It is exactly what Obi-Wan Kenobi meant when he said to Luke Skywalker, "The Force is within you!" In this case it is the force to live life more fully, completely, and healthfully by tapping into our own mind-body connections.

CHAPTER 7

FUNCTIONAL FITNESS: LIVING FULLY FOR A LIFETIME

RICK

Rick came to me with an unusual request but one that was music to my ears. When I first saw him in my office, I was struck by his matter-of-fact tone and the way he asked good questions, listened intently, looked me in the eye, and followed up with an equally penetrating inquiry. But I was also puzzled by why he had come to see me because he didn't seem sick at all. He had an athletic spring in his step and, despite his having gained ten or fifteen pounds over the years, seemed trim and quite youthful for fifty-eight.

"I'll come right to the point, Doctor," he said. "I'm not here because of a pressing medical problem; I'm here because I like the hand I've been dealt and want to be at the table for as long as possible." Rick went on to explain. He had built a long and successful career in one of the largest department stores in New England. He had risen through the ranks until at age forty-eight he had reached his current position of senior vice-president of human resources. He was respected, well compensated, and healthy.

He was also in a position to see or arbitrate most of the human problems in a work force of over four thousand individuals. And his visit to me had been prompted by an event that had happened several weeks before as a result of the sale of his department store to a large chain after fifty years as a family-owned, independent business. Part of the acquisition process involved the downsizing of the work force by 20 percent, and the unpleasant task of terminating managers had fallen to him.

"Two weeks ago I met with Frank, a department manager in his mid-fifties who was being asked to retire," Rick said. "He took it very hard. Frank had been with the company for over twenty years, almost as long as I had. As I counseled him about possible second-career paths open to him, it slowly dawned on me that his options were really limited. While his personnel folder listed his age as fifty-five, everything about him seemed at least ten years older—both physically and emotionally. While he hadn't abused himself, he clearly hadn't taken care of himself. His only real option was to retire. I felt bad for him, but I also vowed that I was never going to let myself get into that position."

This experience crystallized Rick's thinking about what he was doing to assure the kind of longevity and productivity he wanted from the rest of his life. More important, it galvanized him into action. Viewing Frank's plight made Rick take stock of other circumstances in his life. The eldest of four children, he had primary responsibility for the care of his parents, both in their early eighties. They had managed reasonably well in their own home until, at eighty-two, his mother had slipped and broken her hip. After a tumultuous hospital stay she had returned home briefly but was so weakened that she couldn't navigate the one flight of stairs in their tiny home. After considerable agony the family had finally decided that a nursing home was her only alternative. His father, now living alone for the first time in his adult life, was losing weight and thinking poorly. Rick was worried his father would also require institutionalization. At work Rick had watched one colleague die of a heart attack and another retire after three coronary artery bypass grafts. Clearly Rick had reasons to think about his own life, and he was determined to do what he could to maximize both his health and years of independent living.

When I examined Rick, the good news was that he was basically healthy. His blood pressure was an excellent 134/80, his weight of 195 pounds was 15 pounds overweight for his height of five feet eleven, his chest and lungs were clear, and there was no evidence of cancer. His flexibility was somewhat diminished, particularly in his left knee (where he had suffered a football injury in college). His strength was above average for his age, and his reflexes were normal. All his routine laboratory values, including blood work and electrocardiogram, were entirely normal except for a slightly elevated cholesterol level of 220. His functional fitness testing revealed only minor abnormalities: His balance test results and fifty-foot walk time were below average. His exercise tolerance test showed no evidence of coronary artery disease and an average aerobic capacity (VO^2 max) of 34 ml/kg/min for a man his age.

When I saw Rick the next week in my clinic, I was in the happy position of telling him that no evidence of disease existed and we were ready to embark on a program to increase his functional fitness. I gave him a regular walking program supplemented with strength training three times a week and daily flexibility exercises. We worked out a nutritional program that would enable him to lower his fat consumption and cholesterol level and, along with his new exercise routine, help him shed the extra fifteen pounds he had accumulated over the years. In addition, I challenged him to learn a new sport or hobby and take disciplined rest periods, such as weekends off or short vacations with his wife. Rick's grin lit up the small exam room. Not only was his basic health intact, but he had a plan to structure his activities to meet his goal of "being at the table for as long as I can."

When I saw Rick the next year, the changes were apparent. He had lost ten pounds and was 20 percent stronger. He had logged more than a thousand miles of walking during the year and picked up the game of tennis, taking lessons from a local pro. His energy level was higher than when he had been in his thirties, and he had begun considering taking an early retirement from his company to pursue his lifelong entrepreneurial dream of starting his own consulting firm.

Because he had taken control, Rick was functioning at his own peak level, not at some arbitrary level dictated by others around him, by social expectations, or by his own indifference. Instead he was preparing daily to be a full participant for the rest of his life in whatever challenges it might bring.

WHAT IS FUNCTIONAL FITNESS?

In a sense, all fitness activities relate to our ability to function. Yet until we get into our forties and beyond, we often fail to understand the connection. When we're young, we have so much excess capacity in terms of cardiovascular or aerobic capacity and strength and endurance that we tend to treat them as separate, unrelated facets of our lives. We think we'll live forever and unfortunately often conduct our lives as if we will. It's only as we mature that we recognize the interconnectedness of life and the need to live and plan in an integrated way. Functional fitness, in fact, is possible only when we approach living this way.

Stated simply, then, functional fitness is fitness in the service of optimal function. It's using our daily practices and habits to build and maintain the abilities that will, as Rick aptly put it, ensure that we're at the table for as long as possible.

In the previous two chapters I've emphasized fitness in the service of physical and mental health, yet fitness in the service of function is strongly related to good health—and just as important. It's hard to maintain good health and a sense of well-being if your ability to perform the daily tasks that invigorate your existence is impaired. In fact, I believe one of the biggest fears we all share as we face growing older is loss of function and control of our faculties—both mental and physical. Consequently, functional fitness starts becoming an issue for people in their forties and assumes increasing importance every decade thereafter. Just as we all want good health, so we all fear diminished function.

Fortunately there are simple things each of us can do, right now, that will make an enormous difference in our ability to function in the years and decades ahead. That's why I said Rick's request was music to my ears. He had framed the problem correctly. He had recognized that his personal actions profoundly affected his ability to function at the level he deserved and desired. He was willing to take the simple steps to ensure his place at the table for the longest possible time. In this chapter I'm going to show *you* how to take those steps.

AN EXAMPLE TO GROW BY

One of the best ways to start you down the path to functional fitness is to tell you about my friend Ted Phillips, whose approach to living fully can light the way for all of us.

My first formal introduction to Dr. Ted Phillips came about two months after I joined the faculty at the University of Massachusetts Medical School. I was walking to grand rounds when I heard footsteps hastening behind me and felt a tap on the shoulder. "Dr. Rippe, I'm Ted Phillips," he declared as he extended his hand. His formality, while appreciated, was entirely unnecessary, as was the need to introduce himself. Even as the new kid on the block I knew who Ted Phillips was;

everyone knew who Ted Phillips was. He was a towering and legendary figure in the hospital, the doctor whom every intern, resident, and junior faculty member hoped they would one day become. Ted had practiced gastroenterology in central Massachusetts for forty-five years. He had built the largest and most successful practice in the area and was universally revered by patients, colleagues, and the community.

In his late seventies Dr. Phillips had the stride, handshake, and visage of a man twenty years younger. His stamina, clinical skill, and bedside manner were legendary. Even though he had cut back his practice some, he was still likely to be completing rounds at seven or eight in the evening and was often the only senior physician around for interns or residents to ask questions both clinical and personal.

Right now he had something on his mind. "Dr. Rippe," he said, "I saw that you're recruiting individuals for a cardiovascular fitness study involving walking."

I nodded. We had posted signs all over the hospital seeking volunteers. The study was my first major research project as a faculty member, and I was both eager and anxious for it to succeed.

"I noticed that the age cutoff is sixty-nine years old," he continued. "That seems a little young to me. What about us old geezers?"

What followed was a pleasant conversation in which I tried to justify the age range of thirty to sixty-nine on this pilot project while he gently prodded me to consider the effects of walking for people in their seventies and eighties. I finally escaped after Ted had extracted the promise that future research would be more age-inclusive.

Over the ten years I served on the faculty, before moving to Tufts, Ted became one of my closest friends and mentors. What I admired most about Ted was his unfailing optimism and inquisitiveness. He asked me more questions, pushed me harder about theories and findings, and contributed more to my growth as a physician than any other colleague I've ever had.

Ted had been an early convert to the health benefits of an active lifestyle. Early in his career, he traveled to Boston on numerous occasions to hear lectures of the grandfather of American cardiology, Dr. Paul Dudley White. Dr. White, who probably achieved his greatest prominence as President Dwight D. Eisenhower's cardiologist, was a staunch, lifelong advocate of the benefits of physical activity. His speeches in the 1940s and 1950s were met with great skepticism and doubt since most cardiologists of the era saw physical exertion as potentially dangerous. When he told the anxious nation in 1954 that President Eisenhower would recover fully from his heart attack as long as he followed a regular walking program, many physicians thought he was crazy.

But Ted took Dr. White's advice to heart and became one of the earliest joggers in central Massachusetts, often extolling its virtues to his patients. He even ran in several Boston Marathons. In his seventies he switched to walking as his fitness program (hence his disappointment at the age cutoff for my study) and was a fixture at the local Jewish community center, where the indoor track was named in his honor.

Ted was forever accosting me in the hallway to expound his latest theory, talk about a new hobby, show pictures of his latest grandchild, or ask my opinion about a patient or a new study that had just been published. When he cut back his practice by 20 percent in his seventies, he started to take piano lessons. "At seventy-five I was probably the oldest beginning piano student in America," he joked, obviously proud of his accomplishment. When I left the University of Massachusetts, Ted was in his late eighties and still going strong.

When I last spoke with Ted, he was eagerly pursuing plans to surf the Internet. "It's the wave of the future, Jim!" he assured me. Riding the wave of the future with such enthusiasm is something we all can strive for with benefit.

WHAT ARE THE COMPONENTS OF FUNCTIONAL FITNESS?

What has given Ted his admirable longevity and quality of life? Is he lucky? Does he have great genes? In all honesty the answer to both these questions is probably yes. But there's also much more than that. What Ted has accomplished through his natural approach to life was what Rick was striving to achieve through attention and careful planning. Both were using daily practices, habits, and decisions as a means to preserve high levels of function in body, mind, and spirit. This is exactly what anyone can do. Whatever the materials we've been handed by heredity or circumstance, we can use them to the fullest. Remember my patient Galen whose heart damage was so severe that his prognosis was less than a year to live but who, with good practices and habits and a great spirit, lived happily and fully for twelve more years?

As I've seen so often in my medical practice, those people who make conscious efforts to maintain functions at their highest level are typically successful. Those who don't end up like Frank, old before their time, their lives and dreams truncated because their functional level has deteriorated. To put it simply, when it comes to functional fitness—both physical and mental—you must "use it or lose it." And the older you become, the more black and white this reality becomes.

Functional fitness results from using (or losing) three basic and interlocking components: physical, cognitive, and emotional capacities. If we would function at our best and live independently for as long as possible, we must have mobility, stability, and adequate cardiovascular endurance and muscular strength—all attributes of physical functional fitness—we need to stay mentally sharp—cognitive functional fitness—we need to have a sense of well-being or joy in our lives—emotional functional fitness. As we grow older, all these components take on increasing health implications.

THE RELATIONSHIP OF FUNCTIONAL FITNESS AND HEALTH

Functioning at your best and being healthy are strongly interrelated concepts. It's hard to function at your best if your health isn't good, and many of the practices required to optimize function are also ways to optimize health. By the same token, it's impossible to be truly healthy if you're not functioning at your very best. Adequate mobility, strength, endurance, a sharp, inquiring mind, a sense of well-being, and optimism—hallmarks of maximum function—all are needed for optimal health.

I do believe, however, that while there are enormous areas of overlap, there are also subtle differences between maximal function and optimal health. Maybe the best way to describe these differences is to say that maximal function is more related to quality of life—what you experience on a day-to-day basis and the pleasure and fulfillment your life brings you—than is optimal health.

Look at the examples of Rick and Ted. Both were basically healthy, but both wanted and got more out of life than freedom from disease. Both wanted to drink deeply from the cup of life, and both pursued strategies to maximize their joy and quality of life.

Of course, maximal function will mean different things to different people. For some it may mean playing vigorous singles tennis into their seventies. For others it may mean setting personal records in the marathon in their forties or the ability to live independently in their own homes until the day they die. But there are several areas where staying functionally fit as we grow older can make an enormous difference to all of us no matter what our individual goals or definitions of "staying at the table."

Staying mobile

Mobility is perhaps the most important element of functional fitness because it has both a physical and an emotional impact for us. By "mobility" I mean the ability to maintain the unrestricted and comfortable ability to get from place to place, and for most people that means unhindered walking. Yet by the age of fifty, 15 percent of individuals have a significant walking impairment, by the age of seventy 30 percent have impairment, and by the age of eighty over 50 percent of individuals have trouble walking.

Difficulty in walking can have enormous practical, physical, and emotional consequences. I'll never forget what happened to Gloria, one of my cardiac rehab patients who, during a six-month period in her early eighties, became progressively more withdrawn and depressed. Since I could find no cardiac reason for her deterioration, I questioned her closely. She finally told me she had had to give up her walking program because she couldn't walk fast enough to get across a four-lane street in front of her house during the traffic light change. (Most people don't know that traffic light changes are set by the federal government using average fifty-foot walk times for young people.) We arranged a daily ride to a mall walking program for Gloria, and immediately her outlook brightened.

Avoiding falls

Another area where functional fitness is critical is in avoiding falls. Falls in the elderly can have devastating consequences and often signal the end of independent living. Of the 200,000 broken hips each year, 170,000 occur to people older than sixty-five. Falls are, in fact, the sixth leading cause of death after age sixty-five for Americans. Yet falls at any age can be an enormous problem with consequences ranging from broken bones to abandoned fitness programs.

Avoiding falls is a complicated issue. They have to do with balance, reaction time, strength, and a host of sensory issues, such as eyesight and hearing, as well as medical issues, such as number and types of medication. Fortunately many of the physical issues related to avoiding falls, such as balance, reaction time, and strength, are strongly related to one another and are instances where your daily life habits and planned activity programs can make an enormous difference.

While I'm on the subject of falls, let me point out that the fear of falling may be just as inhibiting as an actual fall. I've had many patients in their seventies and eighties who have gradually lost confidence in their ability to navigate their daily terrain and consequently narrowed their lives with both unfortunate medical and psychological consequences. Usually a program of increased activity, cardiovascular fitness, and strength training can make an enormous difference in these individuals' functional level and quality of life.

Keeping the wits sharp

Both cognitive function and emotional well-being are also critical to good health and functional fitness. If we are to live independently for as long as possible, we must be mentally alert and able to accomplish each day's tasks and decisions adequately. I have had patients who have had difficulty returning to their normal lives after major operations because they had difficulty following directions for taking their medicines and carrying out their rehabilitation regimens. Fortunately we have learned that physical and cognitive fitness are interrelated; staying physically fit helps you stay mentally fit and vice versa. We also know that people who are involved in social interests—family, friends, business and community activities—do better and are happier.

HOW TO IMPROVE YOUR FUNCTIONAL FITNESS

The key to improving functional fitness is to remember that daily functioning is a complex process and the factors that contribute to your level of function are strongly related to one another. Not only do the physical factors that constitute function strongly relate to one another, but the physical, cognitive, and emotional factors also relate to each other in a seamless web.

Think for a moment of the wonderful example of health, vitality, and functional fitness that I described in Dr. Ted Phillips. We all know people in our lives like Ted, people who seem to defy the aging process and function at a level that exceeds that of people far younger than they are.

How do these people do it? I don't think there's one factor; rather it's a combination of good health, positive daily habits, optimism, and the willingness to continue to learn and grow throughout their lives. That having been said, there are definitely some specific actions you can take to improve components of functional fitness. Let's look at a few.

Physical functional fitness

Let me list a few terms and concepts: physical activity, cardiovascular fitness, strength, balance, mobility, and reaction time. What do these have in common? These factors all are strongly related to one another as our Advil Fit over Forty Standards research project clearly showed.

The practical implications of these findings are enormous. This research shows that if you want to improve your balance, mobility, and reaction time—all key components of functional physical fitness—you should focus your attention on being more physically active, improving your cardiovascular fitness, and becoming stronger. In other words, follow the programs outlined for these factors in various chapters of this book.

Cognitive functional fitness

When I asked him once why at the age of seventy-five he had started piano lessons, Ted Phillips responded, "When a crop stops growing, it's either cut down or rots, and I'm not ready to be harvested!" Ted was a man ahead of his time. Recent research from both Harvard and Penn State has shown that the best way to retain cognitive faculties is to use them. If you want to remain intellectually alive, live with your intellect.

Thomas Edison once said, "Old age is defined by the period when you stop learning." I couldn't have said it better myself.

My prescription for retaining cognitive function: Adopt new hobbies, sports, and activities. Travel. Ask questions. Learn to play a musical instrument. Surf the Internet. Refuse to stop growing.

One final thought here: The research at Penn State showed that individuals who remained physically active and fit maintained or improved their cognitive functions compared with inactive peers. What's going on here? Improved blood flow to the brain?

Possibly. But I suspect that's a minor factor. Physical activity helps us organize, relieve stress, forces us to learn new tasks and use our minds and bodies (remember the mind-body linkages), all of which are important to cognitive function.

I've seen the power of this in my own life. In my forties I took up both downhill skiing and big-wave windsurfing. In both instances my friends calmly assured me that I had totally lost my mind. Wrong! Not only do I love the challenge of these sports and find both incredibly relaxing (I almost said "intensely" relaxing), but the continued challenge of learning new aspects of these sports seems to invigorate all aspects of learning in my life. My next new sport is in-line skating. I've already purchased the skates and protective equipment. When the snow melts, I'm ready to rock and roll.

As I've said throughout this book, body and mind are one, and the same is true when it comes to maximizing function.

Emotional functional fitness

Emotional well-being and function are strongly interrelated. As I've already stated, my chief recollection of Ted Phillips is his optimism and enthusiasm. A recipe for optimal function includes seeking and gaining the love and trust of others. As noted in the last chapter, studies in both animals and humans show that one of the most dangerous aspects of aging is isolation. Family, friends, volunteer work, laughter, trust: What do these words have in common?

When I was a junior at Harvard University many years ago, I had the privilege of taking Erik Erikson's course on "Life Stages" in the year prior to the great psychologist's retirement. Erikson's theory of development follows people through a series of eight stages of life development culminating in the final challenge of "generativity versus despair." With great courage and candor Professor Erikson described his personal struggle to achieve generativity by living fully and passing wisdom to the next generation, rather than the alternative of lapsing into despair.

Professor Erikson died in 1994 at the age of ninety-one, vigorous and productive until the end of his life. Does emotional health relate to physical health?

SURFING

Several years ago my wife and I were featured in an article entitled "It's Never Too Late for Fitness." Why the title? Because when we met, my wife, who was thirty-five at the time and a television news anchor in Boston, had never been serious about her fitness program. While she maintained basic fitness and the slender figure required of a television talent, she wasn't strong, and her endurance was poor. As part of her commitment to me and, most important, to *herself*, she started a serious fitness program. A year later she was 50 percent stronger and had improved her cardiovascular fitness by 40 percent. She had gained ten pounds of muscle and dropped a dress size. Most important, she felt and functioned better than she ever had in her life.

Is functional fitness important to me? You bet! As I said to the writer of the article, we're starting a family at this late stage in life. That means my children will be teenagers when I'm in my sixties, but I intend to ski their butts off. I want to windsurf in Maui with my wife in my seventies. I intend to be making love to her in my eighties and nineties. Isn't that what life's all about? Fortunately what I do and what you do every day have an enormous impact on whether we're at the table or on the sidelines.

PART THREE

FIT
OVER FORTY
FITNESS PROGRAMS

CHAPTER 8

WALKING (AND OTHER ACTIVITIES) FOR CARDIOVASCULAR FITNESS

WALT

Before going to my clinic, as I reviewed new patients' records, I stopped at Walt's chart. It was thin, containing only a letter from his physician describing Walt's situation and asking for advice. I immediately noticed his age. He was only forty-three years old yet had already survived a major heart attack and was now left with significant angina (chest pain) even with minimal exertion. In a sense his situation was not unusual. As a cardiologist I have seen many individuals even in their forties with significant coronary artery disease.

I knew without reading beyond the first paragraph that he was a cigarette smoker. Unless there was some other significant risk factor, such as an inherited form of high cholesterol, people with heart disease in their forties almost invariably are smokers. I suspected that I would also find him very inactive and probably a little overweight, although his low activity level would now be compounded by his angina. As I walked to the clinic, I thought about how often I saw people in predicaments similar to Walt's and what I might be able to offer him.

Walt walked into my office accompanied by his wife, Sheila, in her mid-thirties, and two of their children who were too young to be left at home. After exchanging a few pleasantries, he came to the point. The heart attack seemed to have come out of the blue, and the ongoing chest pain frightened him. He was dejected that his poor lifestyle—in particular his cigarette smoking and lack of exercise—had caused his problem. He wondered what the future held for him and his family.

We scheduled Walt for cardiac catheterization the next week. When we took pictures of his heart and his coronary arteries, the findings showed significant problems but also held out some genuine hope. The front of his heart muscle no longer moved; it had been killed during the heart attack. The good news was that although damage had occurred, the heart was still pumping with 50 percent efficiency. The artery supplying the damaged section of the heart was entirely blocked off. His other two coronary arteries also had some narrowings. One was 75 percent narrowed, and the other was 50 percent narrowed.

I discussed the findings with Walt and his wife. Our options included coronary artery bypass grafting, angioplasty (the balloon technique to open the two narrowed arteries), and aggressive lifestyle management to stop the progress of his coronary artery disease and possibly even reverse the process. On my recommendation, Walt opted for lifestyle management.

What resulted from this approach was one of those small miracles I mentioned previously. We started slowly so that Walt's body could adjust. After all, it takes time to reverse years of neglect. I added several medicines and adjusted others to relieve his angina. Walt quit smoking and, with Sheila's help, started to pay attention to his diet—particularly keeping saturated fat and cholesterol to a minimum. Most important, he started to exercise. He began to walk every day. At first his walks were short ones—usually a half mile a day. Within one month he was at two miles a day, and by six months three miles a day—the level that he has maintained since then.

Slowly I began to notice Walt change. At one month he was feeling better, his endurance was better, angina less frequent, and mood improved. By three months he had begun to hit his stride. He felt more energy and vigor, had lost ten pounds, and had regained his confidence and joie de vivre. He was talking about the future with anticipation rather than reluctance. He felt he had a future. His angina was mild and occasional.

By six months Walt's transformation was complete. He had lost twenty pounds—back to his weight during college. His angina was gone. He was walking three miles a day. He had gone back to high school teaching, which he loved, and was eagerly awaiting the fall football season and a return to coaching. He was happy and planning for a future that seemed as bright as his smile that day.

"You know, Doc," he said, "in a funny way my heart attack was a blessing. It helped turn me around and finally started living. I feel *better physically* and better about myself than I have at any time in my life."

Ten years later Walt is still angina-free, still walking, still drinking deeply from the cup of life. At the very minimum he has prevented the progress of his coronary artery disease and maybe even reversed some of the narrowings. The only way to know for absolute certainty would be to repeat his cardiac catheterization, and I see no reason to do that. He is a man who took matters into his own hands and made his heart disease part of his past rather than the dominant feature of his present and threat to his future.

WHY IS CARDIOVASCULAR FITNESS SO IMPORTANT?

What made Walt so successful? A number of factors: his determination to succeed, his loving wife, his attention to detail, and, yes, his cardiovascular fitness program. Walt's walking program improved his cardiovascular endurance and, just as important, aided his spiritual recovery. In turn, his spiritual recovery contributed to his recovery from life-threatening heart disease.

Walt's story is by no means unique. Over the past fifteen years I have seen hundreds of people turn their lives around through taking control of their daily habits. Some, like Walt, had life-threatening heart disease, but many others were simply out of shape, feeling too old for their age, and determined to find a better way of life. While their circumstances may have differed, the unifying characteristic that changed their lives was to start and stay with a program to improve their cardiovascular fitness. Improving cardiovascular fitness is the easiest way to lower your risk of heart disease. It is also the best way to increase your energy and your ability to accomplish many tasks without fatigue and to improve your mood and outlook on life. It's the closest thing to magic in medicine that I have ever seen.

Preventing heart disease—a message we
need to take personally

Despite the enormous strides we've made in the past twenty years, heart disease is still by far the number one killer of both men and women. More than one million individuals still have heart attacks every year in the United States, and over five hundred thousand individuals die from heart disease. The tragedy is that many of these deaths are preventable.

My role as a cardiologist trying to save people with heart disease reminds me of a story about a man walking along the banks of a raging river. Suddenly he sees a person being swept along in the current and hears a cry for help. Since he's a strong swimmer, the man dives into the water and after a valiant effort saves the drowning person. As soon as he gets to shore, he hears another person in the water screaming for help. Once again he dives in and manages to struggle back to shore, having saved another person. This goes on a few more times before the exhausted man realizes he's got to get to the root of the problem rather than attempt to drag person after person out of the freezing water. He walks up shore, finds the person who is pushing people into the water, and stops that person.

Staying "out of the water"

When it comes to heart disease, we know what's pushing people into the water: our lousy daily habits and practices. That's where we have to focus our attention. The risk factors for coronary heart disease are well known. The American Heart Association identified three major risk factors as long as twenty years ago: cigarette smoking, high blood cholesterol, and high blood pressure. Within the past few years the AHA added a fourth major risk factor: inactive lifestyle—and that's what the Fit over Forty Walking Program will help you overcome. I will also give you tips on other exercise activities that you can use in conjunction with your walking program (or even in place of it) to achieve these goals.

Let me remind you that taking steps to lower substantially your risk of heart disease takes only a few moments a day. I think lots of people put off doing anything about their good intentions to adopt a fitness program because they think they will have to turn their lives upside down. Not so. An important study conducted by the Cooper

Aerobics Research Institute found that all an individual needed to do to receive a substantial reduction in his or her risk of heart disease was to improve his or her cardiovascular fitness enough to escape being included in the bottom 20 percent of the population.

How much exercise is required to escape the bottom 20 percent in cardiovascular fitness? Moderately brisk walking for about fifteen minutes a day. The Fit over Forty Walking Program will help you escape the bottom 20 percent and climb as high on the ladder of fitness as you want to go.

Of course, before you charge single-mindedly into an exercise program, let me remind you that even though improved cardiovascular fitness is one of the keys to improved cardiovascular health, it is not a panacea. You need to combine your exercise program with proper nutrition, stress reduction, and blood pressure control to lower cholesterol and maintain proper body weight—issues covered (complete with programs) in subsequent chapters. Of course, no one concerned with his or her health whether or not he or she currently has coronary heart disease should ever smoke.

What if you already have heart disease?

The good news is that the same basic message applies. In fact, as Walt's case clearly emphasizes, cardiovascular fitness may be even more important in individuals with coronary artery disease. Improved cardiovascular fitness not only strengthens the heart and the rest of the cardiovascular system but also makes the entire body more efficient. Both these effects are extremely beneficial to the individual with coronary heart disease. The heart becomes capable of more work, and since the body has become more efficient, less cardiac work is required at any given level of exertion. Furthermore, improved cardiovascular fitness lowers the risk of progression of heart disease and, when combined with other risk factor reductions, may even lead to its reversal.

There are eleven million individuals in the United States who have suffered heart attacks or have undergone coronary artery bypass graftings or angioplasties. Many millions more have established coronary artery disease. All these people need to start and stay with a regular program of exercise to improve their cardiovascular fitness.

But let me interject a note of caution here: If you have the signs, symptoms, or other manifestations of heart disease, any program to improve cardiovascular fitness must be done under your doctor's supervision.

WHAT EXACTLY IS CARDIOVASCULAR FITNESS?

Having discussed the whys of cardiovascular fitness, let's take a moment to take a more in-depth look at just what cardiovascular fitness is. At its simplest level, cardiovascular fitness reflects the capacity of the heart and the rest of the cardiovascular system to function properly at any given level of exertion. In practice the concept is a little more complex since in my opinion, it should also reflect your overall cardiovascular health, including your risk of developing heart disease or the risk of the disease progressing if you already have it.

It stands to reason that an individual with a low level of cardiovascular fitness will have difficulty performing even moderate levels of exertion (such as climbing a flight of stairs without getting out of breath), while someone with a high level of cardiovascular fitness will have much more capability to perform even high levels of exertion.

In the laboratory this is exactly what we find. We perform more than one thousand exercise treadmill tests every year in my laboratory on people of every age and fitness background. What we look for on these tests are two things: the individual's level of cardiovascular fitness and early signs of coronary artery disease.

The single best measurement of cardiovascular fitness is called maximum oxygen uptake (VO^2 max), the maximum amount of oxygen you can consume per minute. The concept sounds complicated but isn't. Your maximum oxygen uptake reflects two processes in the body: the capability of your heart to pump oxygenated blood to exercising muscles and the capability of those muscles to pull the oxygen out of the blood. As you exercise, your working muscles demand more and more energy. Since muscles acquire energy by combining oxygen with glucose, glycogen, or free fatty acids, the harder they work, the more oxygen they need to get from your blood and the harder your heart works pumping blood through the lungs and out to the muscles. The fitter your cardiovascular system, the more oxygen your heart can deliver to your muscles and the more they can use.

To determine VO^2 max, then, we ask an individual to exercise at progressively higher intensities, usually on an exercise treadmill, until he or she reaches his or her maximum. Throughout the process we measure oxygen consumption until it peaks. It is this peak that we call maximum oxygen consumption. Some marathon runners or other highly fit individuals may have VO^2 maxes of twenty to twenty-five times their resting metabolic rates while sedentary individuals may be able to achieve only ten times their resting rates, or less, before hitting their maximum.

Although we have sophisticated equipment in the laboratory to perform direct measurements of oxygen consumption, the Fit over Forty One-Mile Walk Test that you took was designed on these principles and is a highly accurate test that gives you an excellent estimate of your cardiovascular fitness.

Even if you never took any cardiovascular fitness test before the One-Mile Walk Test, you have informally used these physiological principles many times to rate your performance. For example, when you climb a long hill or flight of stairs and reach the top out of breath, you might say, "Gee, I sure don't have the wind I used to." But let's say you have to climb that hill or flight of stairs two or three times a day for a week; by the end of the week you'll probably notice that you're reaching the top with more energy and breath. You feel good!

Since in this informal way you've probably experienced how quickly activity or inactivity affects your perception of being fit, it won't surprise you to learn that when a previously inactive person begins a program of exercise to improve his or her cardiovascular fitness, the improvements can be dramatic. Often the individual's VO^2 max will improve 15 to 20 percent over the first three months and an additional 10 percent over the three months after that.

Increased VO^2 max—more energy and less fatigue

The most tangible result of this improvement for most people is increased energy and the ability to accomplish tasks with less fatigue. I have seen it hundreds of times. I remember Sarah, a participant in one of our walking studies, coming up to me to say that she was getting out of bed an hour and a half earlier than before starting her walking program. She had so much energy that she was actually looking for tasks to occupy her before the family awoke. Or there was Marty, who lost ten pounds and improved his cardiovascular capacity over 20 percent during the first three months of his walking. "You should call your program the Better Sex Life, Better Golf Game Walking Program," he exclaimed, pointing out great improvements in his life in both areas.

"I've got so much energy I'm mowing my lawn twice a week, even when it doesn't need it," he declared.

Behind the improved energy—a stronger body

The physiologic improvements that underlie the increased energy come from three sources: improved cardiovascular capacity, increased metabolic efficiency of the muscles, and improved mental outlook. Let's look at each.

As your cardiovascular fitness improves, your heart becomes strong, and its capacity to pump blood increases. This occurs through the process we call physiologic dilatation. The heart actually becomes slightly larger, and that allows it to accept more blood and pump more blood out with each beat. This is very valuable during exercise because with each beat the heart is able to pump more oxygenated blood to the muscles.

Of course, when you are not exercising, your muscles do not need this extra oxygenated blood. However, since the heart has a larger capacity, it still pumps out more blood per beat. Since your need for oxygenated blood when you are resting is low, the heart beats less often when you are at rest than it did before your cardiovascular fitness improved. This is the underlying reason why people invariably experience a noticeable decrease in their resting heart rate as their cardiovascular fitness level improves. And a low resting heart rate is thought to be one factor that contributes to cardiac health. As the great cardiologist Dr. Paul Dudley White once said, "Every heart is programmed at birth for a certain number of beats. The question is do you want to take them at fifty beats per minute or eighty beats per minute?"

The normal resting heart rate is seventy to eighty beats per minute, but individuals who are active in cardiovascular fitness programs can achieve significantly lower resting rates. Even though my running program has decreased over the years, I am still active in a wide variety of cardiovascular fitness activities on a daily basis. I've maintained my resting heart rate below fifty beats a minute for the last twenty-five years. We have tested marathon runners and competitive cyclists with resting heart rates as low as forty beats per minute.

The second adaptation that occurs when your cardiovascular fitness level improves is that your muscles become more efficient. The cells of the muscles contain microscopic structures called mitochondria, which serve as the miniature power packs of the cells and are responsible for combining oxygen with glucose to produce energy. When your cardiovascular fitness improves, your muscles develop more mitochondria and their enzymes become more efficient, allowing the muscles to pull oxygen out of the blood more efficiently.

The third reason people feel more energy when their cardiovascular fitness levels improve is that their mood and mental outlook improve. Exercise has a wonderful calming effect, decreases anxiety, elevates mood, and builds self-esteem, as I discussed in the earlier chapter on mind-body relationships.

HOW EXERCISE HELPS YOU ACHIEVE CARDIOVASCULAR FITNESS

The types of exercise programs required to improve cardiovascular fitness are based on what we call aerobic exercise. "Aerobic" means "in the presence of air," and aerobic exercises are those that challenge and expand the body's oxygen-carrying capacity and systems by having you exercise at levels (60 to 80 percent of maximum capacity) that safely stress or "overload" your system just a little. Your heart, cardiovascular system, and muscles then react to that stress by growing stronger as just described.

The aerobic exercises are characterized by using the body's large muscle groups in a repetitive and continuous fashion because this type of activity generates the necessary levels of stress to get the job done. The wide variety of aerobic exercises includes such common activities as walking, jogging, cycling, swimming, rowing, cross-country skiing, in-line skating, and aerobic dancing.

But how, you ask, do you know that you are working at the right level to achieve the goals you set? For many years, experts have advised that the three characteristics necessary for effective aerobic exercise are duration, intensity, and consistency. That's where the classic prescription of "thirty minutes of exercise, at 60 to 80 percent of maximum capacity, three times a week" comes from. But remember the importance of accumulating physical activity and our continuum of fitness benefits: If you've been inactive, some activity is better than none; if you've been active, then more activity is better than some. Start where you are and build.

I encourage people to do that by putting duration (the time you spend), consistency, and, most important, enjoyment ahead of intensity. For example, walking or stationary cycling at a brisk pace for forty-five minutes is a lot better than fifteen minutes of jogging or nonstop, high-impact aerobic dance, particularly if you are new to exercise.

Of course, many programs, including the Fit over Forty Walking Program, provide intensity levels, usually measured as a percentage of your maximum heart rate (which gives an excellent indication of how hard your body is working), as a guide. I will show you how to use these in a moment but caution you that they are not the most important thing. Working at a level that you perceive as "brisk" as opposed to "easy" or "hard" can also keep you working at the right pace.

DO YOU NEED AN EXERCISE TREADMILL TEST BEFORE UNDERTAKING AN EXERCISE PROGRAM?

I mentioned earlier that it is a good idea for anyone who has been sedentary to check with his or her doctor before beginning an exercise program. But you may be wondering if you need an exercise treadmill stress test to be absolutely sure.

Although cardiologists agree that a treadmill test is clearly indicated as a diagnostic procedure for any individual who has symptoms of heart disease, such as chest, arm, back or jaw pain with exertion, using the exercise treadmill test as a screening device in individuals who do not have symptoms of heart disease remains somewhat controversial, and I recommend that you discuss your specific situation with your physician. In general, individuals over the age of forty-five who have been very sedentary and wish to start a cardiovascular fitness program should strongly consider having a physician-supervised exercise treadmill test prior to starting their exercise program. Younger individuals who have established risk factors for heart disease, such as cigarette smoking, elevated blood cholesterol, or hypertension, should also consider this test prior to starting an exercise program.

THE FIT OVER FORTY WALKING PROGRAM FOR CARDIOVASCULAR FITNESS

Of the many forms of aerobic exercise, I have chosen walking for *Fit over Forty*'s primary aerobic program because I believe that walking is the simplest, most practical, enjoyable, and effective way for most people to achieve improvements in their cardiovascular fitness and establish exercise programs they can stick with for the rest of their lives. Walking is also by far the most common form of exercise physicians recommend to their patients. In a recent survey over 90 percent of physicians recommend walking as the best form of exercise for their patients. All the other forms of aerobic exercise combined were the first choice of less than 10 percent of physicians.

For the past decade my laboratory has been the leading walking research laboratory in the world. We developed the first fitness test based on walking, which has now been taken by millions of people around the world. We have studied walking for all age groups and fitness levels and for a variety of reasons, including improved cardiovascular fitness, weight management, stress reduction, mind-body enhancement, control of hypertension, cholesterol management, and therapy for coronary artery disease. We have started thousands of people on safe and effective walking programs and learned their secrets of success.

All this research and experience have shown that walking is a highly effective, enjoyable, and safe way to improve your cardiovascular fitness. It's my number one recommendation for the vast majority of adults.

An overview of the Fit over Forty Walking Program

On the basis of findings of the Advil Fit over Forty Standards study and a number of previous studies, we have developed the Fit over Forty Walking Program to provide a twelve-week program that is appropriate for your age, sex, and current cardiovascular fitness level as indicated by the Fit over Forty One-Mile Walk Test. Each of the five programs begins at your current level and provides all the steps you need to improve your cardiovascular fitness. At the end of twelve weeks you may retest yourself using the Fit over Forty One-Mile Walk Test and establish a new walking program. Alternatively, you may simply use the mileage and pace established for week 12 to constitute a "maintenance" program for lifelong fitness.

After a brief description of the simple equipment you need and what's involved in a walk session, you'll be ready to determine the correct walking program for you and get started.

Gearing up

One of the great advantages of walking is its simplicity. There are few equipment needs. However, there are a few things you'll need to know.

First, buy a good pair of shoes specifically designed for fitness walking. Many brands are available; however, the key unifying feature is that they are specifically designed for the unique biomechanics of brisk or fitness walking. Fitness walking differs somewhat from regular walking and significantly from jogging. Since fitness walking occurs at a somewhat faster pace than regular walking, the foot and all the joints of the leg, including the ankle, knee, and hip, are under slightly more stress. The shoe should be designed to provide additional support and cushioning.

The biomechanics of jogging are different from fitness walking. In jogging you leave the ground with every stride, and when you land, you land with three to four times your body weight. In contrast, in fitness walking one foot is always in contact with the ground, and the forces remain at one to one and a half times body weight. The soft materials in a jogging shoe required to cushion the higher forces of jogging are not needed for fitness walking and, in fact, make it difficult to provide the stiff sole needed to support the foot properly during the forward rolling motion of the walking stride.

Many excellent brands of walking shoes are available. Whether you buy your shoes in a regular shoe store or an athletic shoe store, look for a knowledgeable salesclerk who can explain the features of shoes designed for fitness walking and help you select the specific brand most suitable for your needs.

Clothing required for fitness walking is also relatively simple. Choose any clothing designed for athletic wear. It should be loose enough to allow for the motions of brisk walking. Wearing layers is a good idea since this allows you to shed outer layers when you get warm in the midst of your fitness walking session. It is also a good idea to own a warm-up suit made with waterproof, breathable fabric or other suitable rain-resistant gear so that your program will not be interrupted by inclement weather.

Step by step through a session of your walking program

Sure, walking's simple. We all do it. But each walking program I will give you will provide specific directions for the following elements in each session to help you get maximum benefit safely and efficiently: warm-up, distance to be walked, pace, time walked, target intensity level (as a percentage of maximum heart rate), cooldown, and frequency (times per week).

Warm-up. To prevent injury (and work on flexibility), you'll warm up with some prewalk stretches. Use the general stretching program in Chapter 11, being sure to stress the muscles of the lower body. You will also want to warm up by starting your walk slowly and gradually increasing your pace.

Distance. The distance you are to walk each session is given in miles. If you're walking on a track or treadmill, distances are easy to determine. If you're walking around the neighborhood, you may want to drive along your favorite route and record appropriate distances for your program. Record distances on several routes for variety.

Pace. The speed at which you should walk is given in miles per hour. If, let's say, you're just getting started (after being very sedentary) and you are supposed to walk 0.5 mile at 2 miles per hour, then you should walk at a pace that will enable you to walk the 0.5 mile in fifteen minutes.

Time walked. This column tells you how many minutes it will take you to walk the recommended distance at the recommended pace.

Heart rate. (percentage of maximum). If you walk each session's distance at the indicated pace, you will achieve the proper intensity indicated in this section. Remember what I said about emphasizing enjoyment, consistency, and duration over intensity.

You may also achieve the proper intensity by maintaining your heart rate in a target heart rate zone that represents exertion levels that are expressed as a percentage of your maximum heart rate. The target heart rates for the five Fit over Forty Walking Programs range from 50 to 80 percent depending on the fitness level.

If you would like to use target heart rate zones as a guide during your walking sessions, you first need to figure your target heart rate zones and then keep track of your heart rate either with a heart rate monitor or by taking your pulse manually.

The procedure for estimating maximum heart rate takes advantage of the fact that our maximum heart rate declines as we age. So to estimate your maximum heart rate, subtract your age from 220 beats per minute. If you are fifty, then 220 minus 50 gives you a maximum heart rate of 170 beats per minute (bpm). To figure your target heart rate zone, multiply your maximum heart rate by the percentage given. For example, let's say you are to walk your 0.5 at 50 to 60 percent of maximum. You multiply 170 by 0.5 (50 percent) to get 85 heartbeats per minute for the low end of your range and 170 by 0.6 (60 percent) to get 102 beats per minute, the top of your range. So you will want to walk at a pace that keeps your heart rate between 85 and 102 beats per minute.

The most accurate way to monitor your heart rate during exercise is to purchase and use a wireless heart rate monitor. We have used these devices in my laboratory for the past ten years and achieved great success with them. Some models allow you to set target rate zones and beep when you stray above or below your zone.

With a little practice, you can also learn how to take your heart rate by feeling your own pulse. To take your pulse manually, you need a watch that indicates seconds. To locate your pulse, gently press your first and second fingers (not your thumb) on your wrist or on the side of your neck just below the curve of your jaw. Count your pulse for fifteen seconds, and multiply by 4 to get your heart rate (bpm). To check that you are walking in your target zone, pause briefly after you are in full swing and check; adjust your pace up or down, and maintain that level of effort until you begin to slow your pace into cooldown.

Cooldown. As you approach the end of your walk, slow your pace to begin your cooldown; complete your cooldown with the same series of stretches that you used prior to the walk (page 121).

Frequency. This tells you the times a week you should walk (or perform an alternate aerobic activity).

Determining the correct Fit Over Forty Walking Program for you

Once you have taken the Fit over Forty One-Mile Walk Test, determining your appropriate walking program is easy. Check your Personal Fitness Profile score for the test to see what your cardiovascular fitness category was: excellent, good, average, fair, or poor. Then consult the Men's or Women's Walking Program, and find the appropriate category for your age and fitness level. You will see that these two parameters place you into one of the five color-coded walking programs: Blue, Green, Yellow, Orange, and Red.

To start on the appropriate walking program for your current aerobic fitness level, turn to the appropriate color program on the next few pages. And don't be blue if you have to start with Blue; this is your first step on that journey to peace and prosperity I promised.

WOMEN'S WALKING PROGRAM CHARTS

	40–49	50–59	60–69	70+
Excellent	Red	Red	Orange	Yellow
Good	Orange	Orange	Yellow	Green
Average	Yellow	Yellow	Green	Blue
Fair	Green	Green	Blue	Blue
Poor	Blue	Blue	Blue	Blue

MEN'S WALKING PROGRAM CHARTS

	40–49	50–59	60–69	70+
Excellent	Red	Red	Red	Orange
Good	Red	Red	Orange	Yellow
Average	Orange	Orange	Yellow	Green
Fair	Yellow	Yellow	Green	Blue
Poor	Green	Green	Blue	Blue

BLUE PROGRAM

Week	1–2	3–4	5	6	7–8	9	10	11	12
Warm-up (min)	5–7	5–7	5–7	5–7	5–7	5–7	5–7	5–7	5–7
Mileage	0.5	0.6	0.75	0.75	0.8	0.9	1.0	1.0	1.1
Pace (mph)	2.0	2.0	2.5	2.5	2.5	3.0	3.0	3.0	3.0
Time walked (min)	15	18	18	18	19.5	18	20	20	22
Heart rate (% of max)	50–60	50–60	60	60	60–70	60–70	60–70	60–70	60–70
Cooldown (min)	5–7	5–7	5–7	5–7	5–7	5–7	5–7	5–7	5–7
Frequency (times per week)	5	5	5	5	5	5	5	5	5

At the end of the twelve-week fitness walking protocol, retest yourself to establish your new program.

GREEN PROGRAM

Week	1–2	3–4	5–6	7	8–9	10–12
Warm-up (min)	5–7	5–7	5–7	5–7	5–7	5–7
Mileage	0.75	0.8	1.0	1.0	1:25	1.5
Pace (mph)	2.5	2.5	2.5	3.0	3.0	3.0
Time walked (min)	18	20	24	20	25	30
Heart rate (% of max)	50–60	60	60–70	60–70	60–70	60–70
Cooldown (min)	5–7	5–7	5–7	5–7	5–7	5–7
Frequency (times per week)	5	5	5	5	5	5

At the end of the twelve-week fitness walking protocol, retest yourself to establish your new program.

YELLOW PROGRAM

Week	1	2	3–4	5	6–8	9–10	11–12
Warm-up (min)	5–7	5–7	5–7	5–7	5–7	5–7	5–7
Mileage	1.0	1.1	1.25	1.5	1.5	1.75	1.75
Pace (mph)	2.5	2.5	2.5	2.5	3.0	3.0	3.5
Time walked (min)	24	27	30	36	30	30	26
Heart rate (% of max)	60–70	60–70	60–70	60–70	60–70	60–70	70
Cooldown (min)	5–7	5–7	5–7	5–7	5–7	5–7	5–7
Frequency (times per week)	5	5	5	5	5	5	5

At the end of the twelve-week fitness protocol, retest yourself and move to a new fitness walking category or follow the Yellow Maintenance Program for a lifetime of fitness walking.

Yellow Maintenance Program

WARM-UP: 5–7 minutes before-walk stretches

AEROBIC WORKOUT: mileage: 1.75; pace: 3.5 mph

HEART RATE: 70 percent of maximum

COOLDOWN: 5–7 minutes after-walk stretches

FREQUENCY: 5 times per week

WEEKLY MILEAGE: 8.75 miles

ORANGE PROGRAM

Week	1	2	3–4	5	6	7	8	9–10	11–12
Warm-up (min)	5–7	5–7	5–7	5–7	5–7	5–7	5–7	5–7	5–7
Mileage	1.25	1.5	1.5	1.6	1.6	1.75	1.75	2.0	2.0
Pace (mph)	2.5	3.0	3.0	3.0	3.5	3.5	3.5	3.5	4.0
Time walked (min)	30	30	30	32	27	30	30	34	30
Heart rate (% of max)	60–70	60–70	60–70	60–70	70	70	70	70	70
Cooldown (min)	5–7	5–7	5–7	5–7	5–7	5–7	5–7	5–7	5–7
Frequency (times per week)	5	5	5	5	5	5	5	5	5

At the end of the twelve-week fitness walking protocol follow the Orange/Red Maintenance Program for a lifetime of fitness walking.

Orange Maintenance Program

WARM-UP: 5–7 minutes before-walk stretches

AEROBIC WORKOUT: mileage: 2.0 pace: 4.0 mph

HEART RATE: 70 percent of maximum

COOLDOWN: 5–7 minutes after walk stretches

FREQUENCY: 5 times per week

WEEKLY MILEAGE: 10 miles

RED PROGRAM

Week	1	2	3	4	5	6	7–12
Warm-up (min)	5–7	5–7	5–7	5–7	5–7	5–7	5–7
Mileage	1.5	1.6	1.75	1.75	1.8	2.0	2.25
Pace (mph)	3.5	3.5	3.5	4.0	4.0	4.5	4.5
Time walked (min)	26	27	30	26	27	27	30
Heart rate (% of max)	70	70	70	70	70	70	70–80
Cooldown (min)	5–7	5–7	5–7	5–7	5–7	5–7	5–7
Frequency (times per week)	5	5	5	5	5	5	5

At the end of the twelve-week fitness protocol follow the Orange/Red Maintenance Program for a lifetime of fitness walking.

Red Maintenance Program

WARM-UP: 5–7 minutes before walk stretches

AEROBIC WORKOUT: mileage: 2.25; pace: 4.5 mph

HEART RATE: 70 percent of maximum

COOLDOWN: 5–7 minutes after-walk stretches

FREQUENCY: 5 times per week

WEEKLY MILEAGE: 11.25 miles

SUCCEEDING WITH CARDIOVASCULAR FITNESS

We've all had the experience of starting an exercise program with the best of intentions only to see our commitment falter when our lives got busier or we became discouraged. It does not have to be this way. There are a few things you can do to fight discouragement before it occurs and maximize the likelihood that you will adopt a cardiovascular fitness program for the rest of your life.

While most of this chapter has focused on brisk walking, there are many other wonderful forms of aerobic exercise. Like many people, I personally find it most enjoyable to mix and match aerobic exercises. This allows me to vary activities from day to day or season to season and keeps my motivation and enthusiasm high. Varying aerobic activities also allows you to exercise different muscle groups and decreases the likelihood that you will develop an overuse injury.

In my own life the core of my program has shifted from running to walking. It would be a rare evening when I am not traveling that my wife and I don't go for a half hour walk together. Nonetheless, I still maintain a regular jogging program of two to three times a week and fill in with stationary stair stepping and cycling.

In practice you'll find what works for you and what fits into your lifestyle. Remember that the keys to maintaining a regular cardiovascular fitness program are enjoyment, convenience, and companionship, so keep these foremost in your mind as you choose your program.

OTHER FORMS OF AEROBIC EXERCISE

If you choose one of the other forms of aerobic activity as the core of your program or use one as variation on a day-to-day or week-to-week basis, you can adapt each exercise to your needs if you use the guidelines given in the walking exercise programs in this chapter. The key considerations are time and intensity.

Each of the walking programs gradually increases distance and pace to produce a slow increase in the number of minutes exercised and the intensity level achieved, based on a percentage of predicted maximum heart rate. If you decide to substitute another aerobic activity for walking, use the minutes of exercise and percentage of predicted maximum heart rate as your guidelines.

For example, if your walking program calls for twenty minutes of walking at 70 percent of predicted maximum heart rate on a given day and you decide to swim or jog on that particular day, use the guideline of performing this alternate activity for twenty minutes at 70 percent of your predicted maximum heart rate. Following this procedure makes it easy to substitute one aerobic activity for another on a daily, weekly, or seasonal basis. (If you skipped over the instructions for determining your maximum heart rate and how to monitor your heart rate during exercise, go back to page 121.)

With this as background, let's look at some of the other forms of aerobic exercise.

Jogging

Jogging is a wonderful activity to improve cardiovascular fitness. Even though I have retreated from my "fanatical" days of jogging, I still derive great pleasure from it and consistently jog three or four times a week for a distance of approximately three miles.

If you are going to jog as the core of your cardiovascular fitness program, there are several issues you'll need to address. First there is intensity. Unless you are already a regular jogger, in my experience, people who start their cardiovascular fitness program with jogging tend to try to go too fast when they begin. Make sure that you keep your heart rate in the 60 to 70 percent of predicted maximum range just as you would if you were starting a walking program. Later, after your cardiovascular system and muscles have become somewhat accustomed to jogging, you can up the pace so that your heart rate is 70 to 80 percent of predicted maximum.

A good general rule of thumb, particularly when you are starting your jogging program (or any other form of cardiovascular fitness program, for that matter), is not to be so out of breath that you can't carry on a normal conversation with the person next to you. You don't need to be able to sing or shout, but you should have enough breath to talk. If you're too breathless to do this, you are exercising too hard. This is by far the most common problem I see when people start a new jogging program or any other program of cardiovascular fitness.

The second key consideration in jogging is injury prevention. Always stretch and warm up before starting, and stretch and cool down following your exercise session. The all-purpose stretches given in Chapter 11 are adequate for jogging or any other form of aerobic exercise and should be performed as part of both warm-up and cooldown.

Of particular concern in jogging is the impact on bones and joints. As I have already mentioned, when you jog you spring off the ground with every step and when you land, you land with the impact of three to four times your body weight. Excellent, well-padded jogging shoes are mandatory to cushion this impact and lower your risk of injury. The clerks at any athletic store should be able to teach you about the feature of the numerous good jogging shoes available and help you select ones that are right for you.

Cycling

Cycling, either outdoors or on a stationary cycle indoors, is an excellent form of cardiovascular conditioning. One particular advantage of cycling is that it is very low-impact since the cycle supports your weight. Thus cycling is a great form of cardiovascular conditioning if you have a previous orthopedic injury. Orthopedic surgeons most often prescribe cycling when they begin the rehabilitation process for an individual who has suffered an orthopedic injury.

A few tips will help you maximize the enjoyment of your cycling program. For outdoor cycling, many people find that it is uncomfortable on their lower backs to ride traditional racing cycles on which they have to bend over. Fortunately the new mountain bikes allow you to ride in an upright position. Major advances in the shifting mechanisms and gearing over the past decade have made mountain bikes easy to use and fun even if you're never going off road. Although I own and use a racing bike and a mountain bike, my recommendation to beginning cyclists is to purchase a street-friendly version of a mountain bike.

The key safety factor for outdoor cycling is *always* to wear a helmet. Most fatalities from cycling accidents are caused by head injuries, and it is estimated that up to 85 percent of these fatalities could be prevented if cyclists wore helmets. Helmets have become very lightweight and comfortable. Around my vacation home in the Berkshires we have great outdoor cycling. We keep three cycles at this house (two racing cycles and one mountain bike) and also have three bicycle helmets. The house rule is that nobody is allowed on a bicycle without a helmet. I wouldn't think of going out to cycle without using mine.

For stationary cycling, make sure that you purchase a comfortable and motivational model. The leading brand over the last fifteen years has been Lifecycle, which we have used and studied extensively in my laboratory for the past decade. A new type that many people find more comfortable than the traditional upright stationary cycle is the semirecumbent stationary cycle. In this type the legs are positioned out in front of you rather than under you and your lower back is supported by a wraparound seat.

One potential negative with both outdoor cycling and stationary cycling is that the exercise is quite specific for the quadriceps muscles of the legs, the muscles in the front of the thighs. Some other forms of cardiovascular exercise employ more muscle groups and may thus be better for total body conditioning.

Stair stepping

I have always thought that the stairs in our buildings represent the most underutilized piece of cardiovascular exercise equipment that most of us have in our daily lives. I am always amazed that people will wait seemingly interminable periods of time to take an elevator for one or two stories when they would have arrived sooner by taking the stairs—and done something good for their heart to boot! I often tell medical students that if they are looking for true solitude, they should take the stairs because no one else is. Don't overlook this great cardiovascular fitness exercise.

Fortunately some wonderful models of stationary stair steppers that are now available can be found in health clubs as well as purchased for home use. The advantage of the stationary stair steppers is that they partially support the body weight and, as a result, are considered low-impact.

I own and use a stationary stair stepper frequently. My only word of caution if you choose this form of exercise is that you purchase a good stair stepper with a recognized brand. Some of the less expensive stationary stair steppers are poorly designed and uncomfortable to use.

Swimming

Swimming is a wonderful form of cardiovascular conditioning with some unique attributes that make it particularly appealing either as a primary aerobic exercise or as part of an overall program of cardiovascular conditioning. First, most swimming strokes provide great exercise to the upper body. Second, since the water supports body weight, swimming is very low-impact. It is particularly good for people who have preexisting joint injuries, arthritis, or orthopedic problems or who are recovering from current injuries.

However, there are two potential negatives associated with swimming: convenience and skill level. If you are contemplating using swimming as a major form of cardiovascular fitness activity, make sure you have ready access to a swimming pool or other place to swim. If you have to travel a half hour each way to get to a swimming facility, it significantly decreases the likelihood that you'll stick with your program. Second, many people don't have the appropriate level of swimming skills to make swimming the major cardiovascular fitness activity in their lives. Unless you were a competitive swimmer at some point in your life, it is a good idea to take swimming lessons when you start your program. Otherwise your level of skill will stop you before your cardiovascular fitness level will and, if you are like most people, you'll become discouraged and quit.

Rowing

Rowing is a great form of cardiovascular conditioning and one of the best total body conditioners available. In fact, when we've tested competitive rowers in our laboratory, they have regularly achieved maximum oxygen consumption in the stratosphere! I remember one Olympic oarsman we tested who achieved a VO^2 max of eighty-four milliliters per kilogram per minute. This was over twenty-five times his resting oxygen consumption and is more than twice the average VO^2 max of the many major-league baseball players we've tested.

Despite the fact that rowing is a great total body conditioner with wonderful cardiovascular fitness benefits, it does have some practical negative aspects. The best form of rowing from both a conditioning and low-injury potential is on-the-water rowing. Yet with very rare exceptions, unless you were a collegiate rower or at some other point in your life acquired training in rowing skills and are fortunate enough to live near a lake or river *and* belong to a rowing club, it is very unlikely that you will be able to maintain on-the-water rowing as your major cardiovascular fitness activity.

Stationary rowers are a reasonable substitute for on-the-water rowing, but in this area you need to be careful. Select a rower that uses as closely as possible the motion that you see oarsmen and women use on the water, with the upper half of your body basically upright. The stationary rowers that require bending at the waist down to the ground on every stroke can be very dangerous for the lower back, and I don't recommend them.

Just as in swimming, rowing requires a reasonable level of skill if you are going to use it as your main cardiovascular fitness activity. An additional issue with rowing is that it carries real injury potential, particularly for your back, if you use poor technique. If you are contemplating using outdoor rowing as your major cardiovascular fitness activity, join a rowing club and get proper instruction. If you're going to use stationary rowing as a cardiovascular activity either at a health club or at home, seek instruction from a qualified fitness professional or personal trainer.

Aerobic dance

I have always been a big fan of aerobic dance for cardiovascular fitness. Almost every year for the past decade I have spoken at the national convention of the International Dance Exercise Association (IDEA). This is the major professional organization for aerobic dance instructors and is filled with enthusiastic individuals eager to learn about the latest information on cardiovascular fitness and health.

One very positive aspect of aerobic dance is that you can join a group or class and get the motivation of exercising with other individuals. There is a downside to this, however. Make sure that you join a class geared to your level of skill and conditioning. You should also try to find an instructor who matches the intensity and movements of the class to the needs, conditioning level, and desires of the students. There's nothing worse than joining an "advanced power funk" class where you learn the latest propulsion jumps and fancy steps when all you really wanted was some moderate-intensity dance to improve your cardiovascular fitness.

You also need to understand before you begin that aerobic dance is almost exclusively a woman's activity. Over 95 percent of individuals in aerobic dance classes are women. No other cardiovascular fitness activity is so disproportionately dominated by one sex. Step aerobics, which many people consider a form of aerobic dance, has attracted more men, but even in this activity the vast majority of participants are women. I don't mention this fact to try to discourage men from participating in aerobic dance and step aerobics. Quite the contrary. I think both are upbeat, motivational forms of cardiovascular fitness activities. I wish more men participated in both.

Step aerobics

When I first saw step aerobics in 1990, I was immediately attracted to it as a wonderful indoor form of cardiovascular exercise. The basic concept of step aerobics is that by lifting your own body weight up and down while stepping up and down on a platform, you can provide an excellent cardiovascular fitness workout with minimal increased stress on the bones and joints.

Even though step aerobics became very popular in the late 1980s and early 1990s, the basic concept of improving cardiovascular fitness by stepping up and down on a platform had been around for a lot longer than that. In fact, this concept was the basic idea behind the Harvard Step Test developed in the Harvard Fatigue Lab in the 1930s and used to test military recruits for cardiovascular fitness for World War II.

If you're thinking about joining a step class, apply the same basic considerations I recommended for aerobic dance. Find a class in which the tempo and complexity of movements are consistent with your fitness level and goals. For most people this means starting with a beginning- or introductory-level step class.

Of course, it is possible to rent or buy home videos to perform step aerobics at home. Many reasonably priced steps are also available to meet any budget, and they typically come with an introductory video. One step platform that I can highly recommend is made by the Step Company. This is the company that invented the original step platform, and it still makes the best one on the market.

There is one other major consideration when it comes to step aerobics, and that is step height. Modern adjustable steps can be easily adjusted to four-inch, six-inch, and eight-inch heights. For virtually every beginner, the four-inch height will be appropriate to start, followed by a slow progression to six inches, and then, for some people, to an eight-inch height. There is no reason to exceed the eight-inch height. In fact, in research performed in my laboratory we've actually shown that going above the eight-inch height is dangerous for people because of potential damage to the knee from the increased height and angle at the knee.

Cross-country skiing

Cross-country skiing is a great form of cardiovascular fitness exercise and a wonderful form of total body conditioning. When elite athletes are tested, the cross-country skiers regularly score at the top in terms of cardiovascular fitness.

In the United States there are virtually no locations where you can perform outdoor cross-country skiing as your major cardiovascular fitness activity all year long and only very selected areas where the snow conditions are favorable for this activity for extended periods. This fact has led to the popularity of stationary indoor cross-country ski machines that simulate the motions of outdoor cross-country skiing.

I am very enthusiastic about using indoor cross-country ski machines as a cardiovascular fitness activity. It's a very low-impact form of activity, and some of the available indoor cross-country ski machines do a good job of exercising both the arms and the legs. There are, however, several cautions that you need to be aware of.

First, in contrast with walking or stationary cycling, the cross-country ski motion is unfamiliar to most people. Be prepared to experience a learning curve over the first few weeks while you get used to using the equipment. In my experience, people who aren't prepared to undergo this learning process invariably give up and don't use their stationary ski machines.

Second, don't expect much improved strength in your upper body. While these machines are advertised as total body conditioners, they still exercise mostly the legs. To improve upper body strength, a very important consideration for most people, you're going to need to engage in some strength training as well, discussed in detail in Chapter 10.

In-line skating

In-line skating has become the most rapidly growing cardiovascular fitness activity of the mid-1990s. It is particularly popular among young people, but it has great potential as a cardiovascular fitness activity for people of all ages. In-line skating uses the major muscle groups of the legs and can provide excellent exercise for improving cardiovascular fitness.

Despite the cardiovascular fitness potential of in-line skating, it does have several drawbacks: the level of skill and balance required and the injury potential.

First, to enjoy in-line skating, you need to acquire enough skill to skate comfortably and—most important—stop! Since, for most people, the skill and motion will be unfamiliar, I strongly urge you to seek professional instruction as you begin this activity.

Second, it is absolutely mandatory that you purchase and wear protective gear when you in-line skate. As I can tell you from personal experience, it is uncomfortable when you fall on concrete when you're learning to in-line skate. Wearing knee guards, wrist and hand guards, and, most important, a helmet will minimize your risk of injury. Fortunately both professional instruction and proper protective gear are available through any major store that sells in-line skates; you simply need to inquire about both.

Having offered these cautions, I remain very enthusiastic about in-line skating. For sheer exhilaration, it's hard to beat. In fact, as I've already mentioned, I have just started in-line skating and anticipate that it will be the next major addition to my personal fitness program.

A FINAL PLUG FOR FITNESS WALKING

As you can see, there are a wide variety of potential activities when it comes to aerobic exercise to improve cardiovascular fitness—enough to fit virtually any interest or circumstance. In practice, for most people the ultimate program they design will probably evolve from a process of trial and error and will almost certainly consist of a variety of forms of cardiovascular fitness exercise.

Even though there are many wonderful aerobic activities available, most people will want to select one activity as the core exercise in their cardiovascular fitness programs and then add activities to spice it up and supply variety.

While the choice of this core activity is up to you, let me put in one last plug for walking. For most people it is the most convenient, comfortable, and practical way to improve cardiovascular fitness, yet it gives all the other benefits achieved by more complicated or difficult aerobic activities.

In the past decade in my laboratory we've studied over three thousand individuals of every age and fitness level participating in walking studies under rigorous laboratory conditions. We've shown that virtually anyone can achieve cardiovascular fitness benefits through walking. In fact, in one study of ten young marathon runners, every single one was able to elevate his or her heart rate into the target training zone necessary for improving cardiovascular fitness just through fitness walking. Oftentimes, in our rush to improve ourselves, we seek complex remedies when simple solutions would suffice.

FINDING PEACE WITH OUR BODIES

With all the wonderful information on the health benefits of improved cardiovascular fitness and all the convenient, fun, and motivational forms of aerobic exercise available, you'd think that everyone would be out there walking, jogging, swimming, or cycling.

Tragically most of us are not—even though we know we should. For too long I think most of us have framed the problem the wrong way. We've turned cardiovascular exercise into a grim and punishing experience rather than a natural, pleasurable part of our daily lives. To see how this can happen we need to look no further than two characters you've met in the first two chapters: Walt and Dr. James Rippe.

Before his heart attack Walt never consistently exercised. He knew he should, indeed often resolved to start, but somehow never found time. It took a life-threatening heart attack before he stopped to see what was happening in his life. Or take Dr. James Rippe, a beginning medical student in the 1970s running forty to fifty miles a week, despite fatigue and even injury, thinking he was somehow improving his health. Even though Walt's and my actions were different, there is a link between them. In both instances we hadn't stopped to listen to the inner voices of our own bodies. Walt's body was telling him it wanted more activity, and mine was telling me to slow down. Once we listened, we changed our lives forever, and for the better.

We need a new way of thinking about our cardiovascular fitness programs, a way that listens to our bodies. You see, we all were born to be "hunter/gatherers." Our bodies are designed to be healthiest and our spirits happiest when we incorporate regular, pleasurable activity into our daily lives. When we do this, we're listening to the wisdom of our bodies.

So I challenge you to think about your cardiovascular fitness program not as a grim and punishing task that is added to your already

stressful life. If you frame it that way, as many people do, you're doom-
ing it to failure right from the start. Rather, view your cardiovascular
fitness program as a natural, enjoyable opportunity to commune with
your body every day. Cardiovascular exercise is God's gift to each of us
as the most reliable way to find peace with our bodies.

CHAPTER 9

STRESS REDUCTION: FINDING INNER PEACE

FRED

I had known Fred for almost ten years. A hard driving, charming guy with the gift of gab and natural sales ability, he had risen through positions of increasing responsibility within the fitness industry to become vice-president of sales for one of the largest health club chains in the United States. Along the way his own fitness program had suffered somewhat as his responsibilities and stress had grown. Now fifty-two years old and twenty pounds overweight, he was lucky if he exercised three times a week. Although his brown hair and beard were now flecked with gray, he still radiated the boyish enthusiasm I had always admired. I always looked forward to our occasional dinners together.

This particular night Fred was his usual animated self, gesturing with his hands as he explained his latest scheme to conquer the fitness business. As he counted out on his fingers the four reasons his current plan couldn't fail, I noticed something unusual about his wrist.

"Fred, why are you wearing a heart rate monitor?" I asked, pointing to his wrist. To the casual observer his watch would have looked like a normal black digital watch, but I recognized immediately that it was a receiver for a wireless heart rate monitor made by Polar. We had been using these monitors in research projects for years and had actually studied them for the past three years.

I knew that if Fred was wearing the receiver on his wrist, he must also be wearing the lightweight transmitter belt around his chest to pick up the electrical signal from the heart and send it to the receiver's digital display.

"It's for stress reduction," Fred replied. "There's a lot of stress on me right now as we enter our major selling season. I found out that I can take little stress reduction breaks throughout the day and nobody even knows I'm doing it!"

He went on to explain. About five years before, at my urging, Fred had purchased a heart rate monitor to help gauge his exercise intensity. Over the years he had noticed an interesting phenomenon. Occasionally, when he was waiting to use a piece of exercise equipment, he would focus on his heart rate. This simple procedure invariably helped relax him, so he began to incorporate it as a regular part of his workout. Both before and after his workout he would sit quietly and make a conscious effort to slow his heart rate by watching the numbers on the heart monitor receiver on his wrist; without fail it calmed him down.

When Fred began having difficulty getting away for his workouts, he thought he'd give the heart rate monitor a try at work. He wore it to work one day, and several times between meetings or while signing correspondence, he made a conscious effort to slow his heart rate. Like magic, it worked. Within a few minutes he was more relaxed and ready to rejoin the battle.

Soon wearing the heart rate monitor became a regular routine—particularly during times of high stress at work. Fred put the chest strap around his chest under his shirt in the morning and wore the receiver as though it were a wristwatch. (Incidentally, most heart rate monitor receivers also serve as digital wristwatches.) All day long Fred was taking mini stress reduction breaks without anyone even knowing it. People just noticed that he was calmer and more productive.

Fred had stumbled on a key to stress reduction. His heart rate monitoring technique pulled him firmly into the here and now, and living in the here and now is the basis of all stress reduction. In addition, by monitoring his heart rate, he was tapping into a natural body rhythm, a practice employed by Tibetan monks for centuries as part of their meditation discipline.

Unfortunately I had to inform Fred that his newly minted stress reduction technique, which he thought was his unique invention, had been discovered centuries before and served as the basis of both modern stress reduction techniques and biofeedback. What he had done, however, had given me a great idea for a research project and a practical way for introducing biofeedback as a stress reduction technique into people's lives.

ALL STRESSED OUT AND NOWHERE TO GO

Fred's example illustrates another feature of the modern world: We have too much stress. I believe that our high stress levels constitute one of the major health risks each of us faces on a daily basis. There is an impressive body of scientific and medical evidence linking stress to a variety of illnesses from heart disease and cancer all the way to the common cold.

Stress is endemic to our modern, fast-paced society. A recent study from the National Institutes of Mental Health found that over 30 percent of adults experience enough stress in their daily lives to impair their performance at work or at home significantly. Work in my laboratory suggests that the number may be even higher. In a survey of over one thousand top corporate executives we conducted several years ago, 53 percent responded that they experienced "quite a bit" of stress in their lives while 17 percent indicated they experienced an "extreme" amount of daily stress. In a more recent survey we mailed to more than a million individuals over the age of forty, of the more than one hundred thousand respondents, 56 percent reported high levels of stress in their lives.

We have a modern plague in our society, and just like the infectious diseases of the Middle Ages, it is killing us—except our plague isn't caused by a microbe; it's caused by stress.

WHAT IS STRESS?

Once, when asked to define pornography, a Supreme Court justice responded, "I don't know how to define it, but I know it when I see it!" Perhaps the same could be said about stress. Although it is frustratingly difficult to define precisely, most of us know it when we experience it.

Over the past twenty years hundreds (perhaps thousands) of articles have been written about stress. Yet perhaps the best and most concise definition of stress comes from one of the earliest books written about it. In this classic book, *The Stress of Life*, written in 1956, Canadian scientist Hans Selye defines stress as "the non-specific response of the body to any demand made upon it."

While very simple, this definition encompasses both key components of stress: a demand (typically external) and a response (typically internal). With this general definition it's easy to see that we face multiple demands (stressors) every day. Perhaps they're issues, such as financial problems, busy schedules, and time commitments, or even physical challenges, such as a cold or a nagging injury. It's not the stressors per se that cause the potential health problems related to stress, it's our *response* to them.

POSITIVE VERSUS NEGATIVE STRESS

Is it possible to have positive stress? Absolutely! In fact, I believe, like many others, that a certain amount of stress is essential for each of us to perform at our best. The concept that stress and performance are related has been around for a long time. Several Harvard professors way back at the turn of the century provided the theoretical basis for this relationship.

In what became known as the Yerkes-Dodson Law, named after the professors who developed it, the relationship between stress and performance is portrayed as a bell-shaped curve. On one side of the curve as stress increases, so does performance. In other words, the right amount of stress can help you do the task at hand better. But at some point, which is different for every person, performance levels off despite increases in stress. Once you pass this point, as stress increases further, performance begins to plummet. You've passed the dividing line between positive and negative stress.

As the Yerkes-Dodson Law postulates, there's an important difference between stress and negative stress. None of us can expect to live a life free of stress. We're surrounded by stressors. It's only when the stress gets out of control or we layer a negative response on top of it that it becomes a problem. There is no doubt in my mind that this relationship is correct. I've seen too many patients, friends, and colleagues reach a point where stress undercuts their performance to doubt there's a limit beyond which stress erodes performance.

Let me give you an example from my own life. I was out of school for six years between college and medical school, a time when, like many young people (particularly in the late 1960s and early 1970s), I explored different jobs before settling on my calling to medicine. But one constant for me during this period was the sport of karate. I had discovered it in my senior year of college and was immediately drawn to its mix of physical and mental discipline. (In a way it was my first exposure to mind-body interactions.) I studied karate every day, eventually achieved my black belt, and even taught it for a few years.

Early in my karate career in a competition I accidentally kicked a fellow student. Fortunately he wasn't hurt—but I broke a toe! If you've ever broken a toe, you know how painful it can be, and you're reminded of your injury with every step. My only consolation was to complain bitterly, hoping at least to gain some sympathy. After listening to my complaints for several days, my karate teacher approached me after class. Rather than offer me the sympathy I was seeking, this wise older man just said. "It is only pain; you worry about it too much."

His simple statement provides a good starting point for a discussion about stress reduction. None of us will avoid pain in our lives. It's foolish to think we can. What we can control, however, is how much we worry about it. The same is true for many other stressors. If we don't control them, our health will suffer as much as our performance.

STRESS AND HEALTH

Abundant medical evidence supports the relationship between negative or uncompensated stress and adverse health consequences. Let's examine several areas where the linkage is particularly clear.

Stress and heart disease

There are multiple links between the head and the heart, and more are being discovered every day. As a cardiologist I never see a patient with established or suspected heart disease without probing his or her emotional life in detail, looking for these links.

Perhaps the most famous established linkage between head and heart was first identified by two California physicians, Meyer

Friedman and Ray Rosenman, in their concept of Type A behavior. In identifying this syndrome, Drs. Friedman and Rosenman described a cluster of emotional behaviors that characterized individuals (typically men) who felt trapped in a constant struggle in life. The struggle was typically seen as unrewarding and complicated by a sense of urgency, frustration, and outright hostility. Drs. Friedman and Rosenman showed that individuals who possessed this cluster of emotional traits were at significantly increased risk for developing heart disease.

Unfortunately the concept of Type A behavior has been widely misinterpreted. Many individuals whom I would call contented hard workers have been misclassified as Type A. As more investigators have explored Type A behavior, it has become clear that it is the hostility component that is particularly dangerous to your health, a concept that Dr. Redford Williams has effectively described in his book *Anger Kills*.

Negative stress can also cause a variety of uncomfortable cardiac symptoms, such as racing hearts or skipped heartbeats, which most people experience as palpitations. There are even instances in which serious cardiac arrhythmias leading to sudden cardiac deaths may be stimulated by excessive stress.

Uncompensated stress can also set off cardiac false alarms. Of the thousands of heart catheterizations I have performed, about 10 percent of individuals demonstrate normal arteries supplying the heart, yet these people first saw me with the complaint of chest pain. What caused their chest pain? In most instances it was stress.

I remember one particular situation that drove this point home. I had been seeing Randy, a forty-five-year-old CEO of a relatively small, publicly held company in central Massachusetts, for about three years for mild hypertension and a slightly elevated cholesterol level. Late one afternoon I received an urgent call from him. He had been having shooting pains in his chest for about half an hour following a heated discussion about a manufacturing problem with one of his senior vice-presidents. He seemed a little short of breath on the phone and reported that he was perspiring. He was obviously distressed. I counseled him to be driven to the emergency room, where I met him.

In the emergency room he already seemed more composed. The chest pains were gone, and he was somewhat embarrassed to have called in the first place. His cardiogram was absolutely normal, and that was reassuring, but I managed to convince him to spend the night in the hospital for observation until I could perform an exercise tolerance test the next morning.

The next morning, to our mutual relief, the exercise treadmill test was entirely normal, and we were able to chalk up the episode to stress. The process of taking his company public had been extremely stressful and the episode with his vice-president had tipped him over the edge to the point that he thought he was having a heart attack.

Stress and emotional well-being

The links between stress and emotional distress are obvious but often ignored. A frequent symptom of stress-related emotional problems is difficulty falling asleep or sleeping soundly. I've also seen stress cause depression, social isolation, and fatigue. The linkage between stress and fatigue is particularly common. While there are some known conditions that can cause fatigue, such as anemia, chronic illness, and even poor conditioning, stress is at the top of my list of possible diagnoses when I see a new patient with this symptom.

Stress and other illnesses

There is evidence linking stress to a wide variety of other illnesses, from cancer to the common cold. For example, in a study conducted by the U.S. Navy, captains who were passed over for promotion to rear admiral had a significantly increased risk of developing cancer over the next year. Other studies have shown that stress is clearly associated with joint inflammation in individuals with arthritis. A recent British study showed that people who were under stress and were exposed to viruses were much more likely to contract upper respiratory tract infections than those who did not report being under stress but were exposed to the same viruses. And the list of stress-related illnesses continues to grow.

How does stress cause physical illness? Although there are many theories and no definitive answers, much of the evidence and speculation centers on the immune system. The immune system fights infection and defends the body against cancers. Abnormalities in the immune system contribute to inflammation in connective tissue and joint disorders, such as various types of arthritis. Various components of the immune system have been shown to malfunction during times of stress, and this malfunction may contribute to a wide variety of illness.

My view is that the immune system is not the only cause of stress-related illness, but it certainly plays a role.

If negative stress is a potent contributing cause of many illnesses, it is also a crafty masquerader. As we saw in Randy's case, stress can mimic the symptoms of heart disease, but it can also masquerade as serious gastrointestinal problems, neurologic disease, connective tissue disease, or simply nonspecific aches and pain, lethargy or fatigue.

The branch of medicine that studies these issues is called psychosomatic medicine. Some remarkable advances have occurred in this area, yet sadly many physicians either are unaware of these advances or don't believe in them. All too often I have seen physicians launch expensive, time-consuming, painful, and ultimately futile wild-goose chases looking for a physical cause for symptoms that turn out to be stress-related.

On the bright side, stress reduction and the mind-body techniques hold great promise as components of therapy. Norman Cousins wrote of his experience "laughing himself well." What he was really telling us about was the body's innate power to heal itself. I always tell patients their hope and optimism are God's great medicines and never to lose them. We've also developed some stress reduction techniques to get our minds working for us rather than against us.

THE POWER OF LISTENING TO YOUR HEART: STUDYING ONE STRESS REDUCTION TECHNIQUE

As I mentioned, Fred's great idea to use his heart rate monitor for stress reduction unfortunately wasn't something he could patent and sell for a million dollars. All he was really doing was applying a biofeedback technique to stress reduction. But the bottom line was that it worked for him, and I thought it would work for others.

With this concept in mind, we recruited some highly anxious individuals (defined by a standard battery of psychological tests) to participate in a simple experiment. Forty were given wireless heart rate monitors and taught how to use them. Each was instructed to find ten minutes a day in a quiet environment, put on the heart rate monitor, and consciously focus on heart rate, trying to lower it. The other forty were asked to change nothing about their lives. We studied all eighty with a battery of psychological tests, looking at anxiety, stress, mood, and quality of life both at the beginning of the study and again after twelve weeks.

The results were dramatic. After the very first session the individuals in the heart rate monitor group experienced significant reductions in their anxiety. At the end of the twelve weeks they had substantial reductions in anxiety and tension, elevations in mood, and improvements in quality of life. All from ten minutes a day of listening to their hearts! When we repeated the tests at the end of twelve weeks, these individuals no longer scored in the "anxious" category. They had dropped their stress levels to "average."

Why did these people succeed? Because they discovered the simple biofeedback technique of paying attention to their heart rates, which pulled them into the here and now, and living in the here and now is the key to stress reduction. When you focus on the present, rather than the deadline you missed yesterday and the one coming up next week, you take control of the many stressors that can affect your life.

THREE PRINCIPLES OF STRESS REDUCTION

Over the years I have had the pleasure of caring for many top executives and athletes. These are individuals who live or die by their performances. And by the nature of what they do they must overcome intense pressure. Often I've engaged them in conversations about stress reduction. While specific answers have varied, some general principles seem to apply to most of these highly successful and "stress-hardy" individuals. Here are three principles they share:

1. Seize the day.
2. Get out of your own way.
3. Make a personal play.

Let's look at each.

Seize the day

This is my way of saying, "Live in the present." A major stress that people put themselves through comes from regretting the past or fearing the future. Without exception the stress-hardy people I've treated have found ways of pulling themselves consistently into the here and now. This, of course, is the essence of the heart rate monitoring experiment I just described, but many individuals have found other techniques.

One of my patients, a senior vice-president of a local Fortune 500 company, told me that he made a conscious effort not to dwell on a problem for more than an hour or two. "If I haven't solved it in that period of time, I consciously put it on the shelf to get some distance," he confided. "Usually when I come back to it, my head is clearer, and I have some perspective."

Get out of your own way

Don't layer additional negative thoughts on top of the normal stresses and strains we encounter in our daily lives. Remember, it's typically not the stress itself that causes the problem; it's our reaction to it.

Make a personal play

This is a reminder to develop a specific strategy to handle stress; don't just leave it free-floating. Without exception the stress-hardy people I've cared for and studied have made specific personal plans for how to handle their stress. While these plans vary widely from exercise to meditation to regularly scheduled vacations and family times, the unifying feature is the presence of a specific and detailed plan to handle the stress that we all inevitably encounter. In the next section you'll learn some of the strategies I believe can be helpful.

PRACTICAL STRATEGIES FOR STRESS REDUCTION

Here are some of the most effective ways I've found to help eliminate stress. Some of these concepts come from my own life and others from patients I've cared for or from research subjects in various studies in my laboratory. In practice some of these strategies may work better for you than others, or you may wish to combine several. I've seen them all work as highly effective stress reduction techniques.

Exercise

No surprise here! Aerobic exercise lowers anxiety and improves mood. As I discussed in the last chapter, slow walks work as well as vigorous runs. The stress-reducing benefits are reliable and immediate.

My advice to beginning exercisers: View your exercise program as primarily for your mind and only secondarily for your body. And be careful about intensity level. Remember, stress reduction benefits come even from slow walks. In my experience, the most common mistake made by most beginning exercisers is to exercise too vigorously. This may actually increase their stress level rather than reduce it.

Listen to your heart

The wireless heart rate monitor technique described earlier in this chapter is reliable, effective, and simple to use. It took people only ten minutes a day to reduce their stress dramatically. The power of this technique comes from using biofeedback and natural body rhythms to pull you firmly into the here and now.

The following technique, based on the research study just described, is adapted from the Take Ten Stress Reduction Program that I developed for Polar Electro, Inc.

Before Each Session
1. Perform your stress reduction session in a quiet location and comfortably seated. Since certain factors can affect your resting heart rate, avoid performing your session immediately after strenuous exercise, a large meal, sitting for a long time, or less than an hour after consuming caffeine (coffee, cola, tea, chocolate). Performing your session at the same time and location every day may be convenient but is not mandatory.
2. Adjust your heart rate monitor and belt properly. Make sure the readings on your monitor are typical for you.
3. Record your heart rate, mood, and stress level immediately before the session.

During Each Session
1. To begin, relax and concentrate on your heart rate readings on your monitor. You may find it helps to focus on the here and now by repeating to yourself such phrases as "down, down, down" or "lower, lower, lower."

Optional techniques: Adding one of the following to your observation of your heart rate may enhance your session: listening to soothing music; paying attention to slow, somewhat deeper-than-normal breathing; visualizing pleasant scenes or events; progressively relaxing every muscle group starting with the foot muscles and moving toward the head.

2. It is okay if your mind starts wandering. You may occasionally fall asleep. If you do, just continue your ten-minute session when you wake.

3. Do not expect to see a dramatic drop in your heart rate. If you try too hard to lower your heart rate, it may actually go up. Simply relax and concentrate on your heart rate readings. Do not become frustrated if your heart rate does not go down.

After Each Session

1. Record your heart rate, mood, and stress level immediately after the session. Also record how you feel and any other general comments.

2. You may want to sit for a few more minutes before getting back to your schedule.

That's all there is to it. If you are like most people, you'll find that your stress level drops and mood improves following the first session. But remember that the greatest benefits come over longer periods, such as the recommended twelve weeks and beyond.

Take time out

Getting away from stressors, even for brief periods of time, is an effective stress reduction technique. Phil, a senior-vice president in a large manufacturing firm, told me it was the key to maintaining his sanity. "It took me years to discover it," he said, "but the key to maintaining your equilibrium is disciplined periods away."

By "disciplined periods away" he meant regularly scheduled breaks from the daily stresses that can wear you down. Those periods might range from a solid week's vacation when you don't call the office to an evening when you admit you're overtired and plan to go to bed at 10:00 P.M. to assure a solid night's sleep.

For some people even the fifteen to twenty-minute daily walk that they do for cardiovascular fitness or weight management becomes an all-important respite from their daily stress. Margaret, a fifty-two-year-old mother of four who joined one of our weight management programs, told me that her half hour daily walk had become the highlight of her day and a guaranteed stress reducer. "For the first time in twenty years I was taking time to do something for myself," she said. "I had always thought that would be selfish. But my family felt exactly the opposite. Sometimes when I was cross with my son, he'd say, 'Mom, it's time for you to go on your walk!'"

Get outside

Now I recognize that it's not that easy for many people to get outside on a regular basis, and sometimes the weather gets in the way, but I strongly recommend it. The outdoor environment possesses magical stress-reducing properties. Maybe it's the connectedness we feel or the sense of timelessness as we walk along a riverbank. Or it's the sheer beauty of watching the leaves turn color in the fall (can you tell I live in New England?) or even watching the lazy snowflakes falling silently to the ground. Something about being in nature taps into the mind's innate ability to calm itself.

Share

The importance of family and friends is frequently overlooked as a powerful stress reducer. Sharing thoughts, feelings, hopes, desires, and frustrations helps put them in perspective. My patients with strong family and community ties invariably do better than those who keep to themselves.

FINDING PEACE WITH OURSELVES

If cardiovascular fitness is finding peace with our bodies, and mind-body interactions help us find peace with our spirits, then reducing our stress is our way of finding peace with ourselves and our circumstances.

Let's go back for a moment to the distinction between stress and negative stress. While we may try to minimize our troubles and improve our lot in life, none of us will lead stress-free lives. In fact, it's probably not *desirable* to be entirely free from stress. Sometimes stress can help us grow and bring out our best. It is when we compound stress with a negative reaction to it that both mental and physical difficulties arise. That's when stress erodes our daily performance, happiness, and health.

If I've done my job in this chapter, I hope I've given you a framework and some specific tools to lower stress in your daily life. Once you do this, you've taken a major step toward finding peace with yourself and your environment—another bridge on our journey.

CHAPTER 10

GETTING STRONGER: PROGRAMS TO BUILD MUSCULAR FITNESS

MARTIN

Martin had a specific agenda in mind. A fifty-five-year-old dentist, he had signed up for one of our strength-training programs because, he said, "I've always regarded myself as young for my age, and lately I don't feel that way." He went on to explain that after a hard day of yard work on the weekend, a couple of vigorous sets of tennis, or even a hard day of standing on his feet doing dental procedures at his office, he could barely crawl out of bed the next morning. "I'm only fifty-five years old, and I shouldn't be this tired!" he declared. "Maybe I need to get stronger."

Although his physical performance at both work and his recreational pursuits troubled him, the episode that pushed Martin into action occurred when he lifted his three-year-old granddaughter at the end of an outdoor play session. Though he'd picked her up a thousand times before, this time he felt something pull in his back. As he carried her back into the house, his lower back was beginning to hurt. Two hours later he was in agony and his back was starting to stiffen up. By the next morning he couldn't get out of bed.

A trip to our emergency room fortunately ruled out the diagnosis of a slipped disk but confirmed my suspicion that he had pulled a muscle in his lower back. The stiffness and pain he was experiencing were not just from the muscle pull but from all the other muscles of the back going into spasm because of the injury. I gave him muscle relaxants and painkillers and told him to stay off his feet as much as possible until his symptoms went away. Martin had to close his dental practice for a week, and it was another week after that before he felt normal. When I saw him in my clinic the next month, we had a detailed discussion about what to do. Obviously the episode had been miserable for him, and he was eager to do anything he could to prevent a recurrence.

I explained to Martin that although he was aerobically fit, he wasn't strong enough. Despite an aerobic conditioning program that consisted of his walking two to three miles three times a week, the muscles of his upper body had grown weak from disuse, and weak muscles become stiff and prone to injury. I recommended that he join one of our strength training research projects to improve his musculoskeletal fitness.

Six months later, when I saw Martin back in the clinic, the results were dramatic. He had participated in a twelve-week strength-training study in my laboratory and then continued his strength-training program at a local health club. During the twelve-week study his overall muscular strength had improved 30 percent. In the next twelve weeks he increased his strength another 10 percent. Without changing anything else in his life, he had managed to lose the ten extra pounds that had accumulated in his forties and fifties. He was playing the best tennis of his life, getting to balls he had previously not even tried for and serving with new confidence and authority. Most important, he was doing all the things in his life that he wanted to without excessive fatigue or soreness. He looked and felt great and radiated the pride of someone who had achieved an enormous breakthrough. Over the past few months he had grown accustomed to people complimenting him and asking for the secret of his success. His reply: "I got strong!"

DISCOVERING THE BENEFITS OF STRENGTH TRAINING

Martin's story is not unique. In fact, his results are almost exactly what I expected when I started him on a well-structured, progressive program to improve muscular fitness. I've seen this type of progress and pride in hundreds of people who have participated in our strength training studies. I've seen it in my own life.

As I've already told you, I have been an avid aerobic athlete virtually my entire adult life. While my running got a bit excessive in my twenties and early thirties, I was committed to cardiovascular fitness and remain so today. Muscular strength and fitness were a whole different kettle of fish. Like many aerobic athletes, I thought I was pretty fit and saw no reason to add strength training to my regimen. Anyway, I didn't really know much about it and thought I didn't have the time.

All this began to change in my early forties. I am an avid recreational athlete. I big-wave windsurf in Hawaii, ski in Utah and Colorado, and play competitive tennis at the club level. Unlike Martin's episode, it was not one event but a series of smaller things that got me started on a regular strength training program. I found that I wasn't able to keep performing the sports I loved at the level I wanted to. I also found that muscle soreness was getting in the way, particularly at the beginning of ski season or for the first few days of a windsurfing vacation. I also started to experience a series of nagging injuries ranging from hamstring and other muscle pulls to my first bout of tennis elbow and a slightly torn cartilage in one knee. About this time triathlons were becoming popular, and a number of my recreational athlete friends were preparing for them with a new concept in training that they called cross training, combining strength training with aerobic conditioning. I was also beginning to see some of the early studies in the medical and scientific literature about the benefits of strength training. For all these reasons I decided to start a personal strength training program.

I'd like to report to you that it was love at first sight, but it wasn't. I was working with a good trainer who helped me learn proper technique and gave me realistic expectations about progression, but I still found strength training, well, painful. I was asking muscles that had grown soft from years of relative disuse to perform tasks they weren't used to. Being somewhat sore became a daily fact of life for me for the next few months.

Fortunately, supported by the encouragement of my trainer and my personal commitment to stick with this new exercise regimen for a minimum of six months before making any permanent judgments, I made it through the first few months. I don't want to paint this as a miserable experience, however. After several weeks the muscular soreness was clearly diminished, and even at that early juncture I could feel myself getting stronger. Over the first six months I improved the strength of most of my major muscle groups by at least 50 percent. Most important, my strength training program had become a central feature of my overall fitness routine, and I looked forward to the three sessions each week.

Eight years later I'm still strength training three times per week. Occasionally, when I am traveling, I'll miss a session or two, but my muscles are so used to the training that I begin to feel uncomfortable if I go for more than three or four days without a strength training session. I am now in a maintenance mode in my strength training regimen. I made the decision after the first six months that I was nearing my genetic potential for strength and didn't need any more for the recreational sports I enjoyed or the other activities of my daily life.

I am still active in windsurfing, downhill skiing, and tennis, and while it's hard to be objective about one's own performance, I think my level of skill and performance has improved over the past eight years. I know for certain that my level of "day after" soreness has diminished, and (knock on wood) I haven't had a significant muscular injury for the past eight years. I not only believe in the science of supporting the multiple benefits of regular strength training but have also seen its benefits in the lives of my patients and in my own life.

STRENGTH AND HEALTH

The medical and scientific evidence supporting the multiple links between muscular fitness and good health has rapidly accumulated over the past decade. This literature is now so overwhelming that in 1990 the American College of Sports Medicine revised its exercise recommendations for the first time in more than a decade to advise every health-conscious adult to add regular resistance strength training to his or her fitness program. The American College of Sports Medicine (ACSM) is the leading organization of exercise physiologists and sports medicine doctors in the world. While cardiovascular fitness exercise remained the core of the ACSM recommendations, strength training was now considered almost as important—and I agree.

Regular strength training offers a number of health benefits, including the following:

The preservation or actual increase of lean muscle tissue

This is the major benefit cited by the ACSM and critical not only to the activities of daily life but also to lifelong weight management (a benefit I'll discuss more fully in a moment).

Maintaining or increasing functional fitness as we age

Strength training is one of the most important potent antiaging activities ever invented. As I've already mentioned, in our twenties and thirties we have so much extra muscular capacity that we don't even recognize that we need to take action to preserve it. Yet we do. Failure to keep our muscles fit becomes an increasing health risk the older we get. Poor muscular fitness starts to show up in our forties and fifties, as it did for Martin and me, but by our seventies and eighties it can be an enormous health risk and a major contributor to the end of independent living. I firmly believe that poor muscular fitness plays a major role in the high incidence of falls and hip fractures in the elderly. Hip fractures cost the nation over thirteen billion dollars a year. On a personal level a hip fracture can spell the end of independent living or even death.

Fortunately, when it comes to muscular training, it's never too late to begin. In a series of incredible studies, researchers at Boston University have shown that individuals even in their eighties and nineties can achieve dramatic increases in muscular strength from safe, structured programs of muscular strength training. Most important, these strength gains are accompanied by improved functional capacity, a key health consideration for anyone over seventy.

Promoting bone density and slowing osteoporosis

Muscular strength training can also play a crucial role in slowing the process of osteoporosis. In a study from Tufts University published in 1995, individuals in their seventies who participated in strength training three times a week for a year achieved dramatic increases in their bone density. In addition, their strength skyrocketed, their muscle mass increased, and their balance significantly improved. They got the best of both worlds. Not only were their bones stronger, but their risk factors for falls and ensuing fractures decreased.

Beyond these, the list of health benefits for regular muscular strength training continues to grow.

STRENGTH TRAINING AND WEIGHT CONTROL

Strength training is both one of the most important components of a comprehensive program for weight loss and one of the most effective things you can do to prevent weight gain in the first place.

Why is strength training so effective for weight management? Because it is so effective at helping to preserve your lean muscle tissue and the *only* effective way to increase lean muscle tissue. Maintaining muscle tissue is critical to weight maintenance because it is the most metabolically active tissue in the body; in other words, it burns the most calories.

A good way to think about this is to view your body as analogous to a car. Your fat tissue is like the trunk of the car—critical for storage but really just along for the ride. The lean muscle tissue is analogous to the car's engine. It burns the gas (in this case calories) and provides the power to get from one place to another. The bigger the engine, the more gas the car can and does burn. The larger your lean muscle mass, the larger the number of calories your body burns, both at work and at rest, and the larger the number of calories burned, the less likely you are to have excess stored as fat.

Unless we are active during our adult lives, our bodies slowly lose muscle tissue. The body interprets inactivity as a state requiring smaller muscles and responds accordingly. After the age of thirty an inactive person loses about a half pound of lean muscle tissue every year. This may not seem like much, but over a decade it adds up to five pounds of lean tissue, which may represent 2 to 4 percent of the total amount. Over the decades this really begins to add up. Imagine periodically reducing the size of your car's engine 5 percent. After a while its power would be noticeably diminished, as would its capacity to burn gas. As your body's lean muscle decreases, so does your ability to burn calories, and unless you decrease your food intake, the inevitable result is weight gain—the dreaded and very common middle-aged spread. We've all known people who attributed their weight gain in middle age to slow metabolism. In a sense they're making the correct attribution. As their lean muscle has declined, so has their "metabolism" since they are capable of burning fewer calories.

In contrast, consistently active people typically are better able to maintain a healthy weight and avoid weight gain with less attention to controlling their food intake because their aerobic activity has allowed them largely to avoid the decrease in lean muscle tissue associated with inactivity. But these individuals may also start to gain weight if their activity level falls even a small amount. I'm often asked by runners and walkers who have gained five to ten unwanted pounds in their forties and fifties what they should do to get rid of them. My advice is always the same: Aside from paying closer attention to their food intake (both portion size and percentage of calories from fat), they should start strength training.

There's one other compelling reason to strength train as a weight control measure, particularly during periods of weight loss. Unless you strength train during weight loss, some of the weight you lose will be lean tissue and you will get *weaker*. But if you strength train during weight loss, you can actually increase your lean tissue, thus increasing your ability to lose weight while you also become stronger.

Claudia, a fifty-three-year-old school administrator who participated in one of our exercise and weight loss studies, provides a great example of this benefit. Over the years her weight had slowly crept up to the point where she was about 30 percent over her ideal body weight and her body *fat* level registered at an unhealthy 32 percent. She was assigned to a group that followed a low-fat diet combined with stationary cycling on the Lifecycle and regular strength training. She was initially reluctant to participate in the group because she thought the exercise would make her tired and even increase her appetite. The strength training in particular scared her because she was afraid she would either get injured or bulk up with unattractive muscles. After some assurances from me that none of her fears was going to happen she finally agreed to "give it a try."

Sixteen weeks later she was like a new woman. "I feel stronger and more fit than I've ever felt in my life," she exulted. The fact that she had dropped two full dress sizes to a size ten almost didn't matter to her. What she noticed was that she felt better than she ever had in her adult life. Her laboratory measurements showed why. She had lost fifteen pounds of fat, while gaining two and a half pounds of lean muscle tissue. Her aerobic capacity had improved 17 percent, and her upper and lower body strength had surged an average of 28 percent.

I'll have much more to say about healthy weight loss and lifelong weight management in Chapter 13. For now, suffice it to say that strength training is a key to any optimum lifelong weight management program.

OTHER REASONS TO STRENGTH TRAIN

In addition to the health benefits of strength training I've already outlined, there are a host of other important reasons for improving your muscular strength and endurance. Let me highlight a few of them.

Injury prevention

Regular strength training is one of the most effective ways of minimizing your risk of muscular injury or injury to the bones and joints. Strong, well-conditioned muscles are healthy muscles, which resist injury. Strong muscles also support and nourish bones and joints and hold them in proper alignment. Weak muscles are unhealthy, stiff muscles and much more prone to injury.

I've already described how both Martin and I used our strength training program both as a response to an injury (or, in my case, multiple injuries) and as a preventive measure to reduce the risk of future injuries. An even more common scenario occurs in individuals whom I call weekend warriors. These people remain inactive all week long, then, when the weekend arrives, don their athletic armor for a recreational sporting joust. All too often the result of these encounters is a significant muscle pull or joint injury. Their usually inactive muscles simply cannot respond to the sudden demands of the athletic competitor. As much as I hate to say it, it is probably safer *not* to play sports on the weekends if you are inactive during the week.

Another variant of the same problem is the avid runners, walkers, or aerobic dancers who develop low back pain as a result of their activity or pull a muscle cleaning the garage or clearing brush on the weekend.

This problem can affect even high-level athletes. I remember an all-star major-league baseball player whom we tested for several years in my laboratory. He was an enormously gifted athlete, yet he had an absolute aversion to off-season conditioning programs. Despite our urging, he refused to run and strength train in the off-season.

Unfortunately he ended up suffering a series of muscle pulls and other injuries that cut short a potentially brilliant career. Bad luck? Maybe. But poor conditioning also played a role.

In all these situations an ounce of prevention would have been worth a pound of cure, and the ounce of prevention would have been a strength training program used as a technique for injury prevention.

Improved physical capacity

Strength training is a great way to improve the capacity of your muscles to perform work. Just as aerobic exercise improves your cardiovascular systems capacity, so does strength training improve the overall capacity of the muscles, and that allows you to accomplish more work with less fatigue. That's exactly what Martin experienced when he found, after his strength training program, that he was able to navigate through a busy day on his feet treating patients and still have loads of energy left over for evenings with his family.

Improved physical appearance

There is no question that regular strength training improves physical appearance. Part of the reason that both Martin and Claudia felt so much better was that in addition to having more energy, they looked better and people noticed.

Research in my laboratory and many others has consistently demonstrated improvements in mood and self-esteem for people who strength train. People who are strong feel better about themselves. The improved physical appearance that follows strength training comes, in my opinion, from the fact that strong, healthy muscles simply look more attractive. You feel more energy, and you feel better about yourself. Surprisingly, energy and self-esteem are two key components of physical beauty. How you feel about yourself and present yourself often translates into how attractive other people find you.

Please understand that I'm not talking about body building and the narcissism that often accompanies that activity. I'm simply talking about the fact that strong muscles look better—and they don't have to be bulky to be strong. In fact, most people over the age of forty who strength train will notice dramatic increases in strength with rather small increases in the size of muscles. In those over the age of forty most of the increased strength comes from increased efficiency of healthy muscles rather than increased size.

Improved physical performance for sports and daily activities

As every major athletic team around the world has discovered, strength training is a key to athletic performance, and this is just as true for the recreational athlete as for the professional or elite competitor. It used to be thought that strength training resulted in bulky, dysfunctional muscles. Modern strength training techniques have eliminated that as a problem. If you are a recreational athlete and want to add five miles per hour to your tennis serve, twenty-five yards off the tee to your drives in golf, or improve your performance in and enjoyment of any report you play, regular strength training is for you.

The reason why strength training is so effective for physical performance lies in three related concepts: strength, power, and endurance. Let me briefly define each.

Strength is the maximum amount of weight that your muscles can lift. An individual who can lift a hundred-pound barbell is twice as strong as the person who can lift only a fifty-pound weight.

Power is the combination of strength and speed. A golfer who can drive the ball 250 yards is twice as powerful for that shot as the individual who can drive only 125 yards. Both may be equally strong, but one is able to generate more club speed through the ball.

Endurance relates to the number of repetitions of an activity that a muscle can perform before becoming fatigued. The person who can step up and down a step platform for thirty minutes during a step aerobics class has twice as much muscular endurance as the individual who is wiped out after fifteen minutes.

In practice all three of these concepts—strength, power, and endurance—are related, and all are important not only for athletic performance but also for the activities of daily life. The three concepts are related to the health and strength of your muscles. The Fit over Forty Upper and Lower Body Strength Tests that you took earlier test both muscular strength and endurance, and the strength training programs found at the end of the chapter are designed to improve muscular strength, power, and endurance.

Mental benefits

As I've already suggested, the benefits that come from strength training are mental as well as physical. People who are strong simply feel better about themselves. Knowing that your muscles are conditioned to perform the tasks you ask them to do is very important to confidence, and confidence, mood, and self-esteem are clearly related to one another.

In our weight loss studies we've shown that individuals who don't strength train often get weaker during weight loss, and this increased weakness is often accompanied by depression. No wonder so many people find it difficult to stay on diets. Strength training during weight loss eliminates the vicious cycle of weakness leading to fatigue and depression.

While, in my experience, the mental benefits associated with strength training are slightly different from those associated with cardiovascular fitness activity, they are just as real. In both instances view your exercise as an activity that is just as beneficial for your mind as for your body.

THE FIT OVER FORTY STRENGTH TRAINING PROGRAMS

On the basis of data from the Advil Fit over Forty Standards and a number of other studies, we have developed two Fit over Forty Strength Training Programs to provide a twelve-week program that is appropriate for your age and current strength and endurance levels as indicated by your results on the Upper and Lower Body Strength Tests. You may choose either program, both of which are appropriate for both men and women.

Program I is designed to be performed at home using calisthenics and, if you wish, adding hand and ankle weights as you progress. I strongly recommend this program for all individuals who are just beginning strength training, and it is highly appropriate for individuals of any strength and endurance level. Program I requires no special training, can be done safely by yourself, and requires little equipment.

Program II is designed for use with free weights and/or machines and requires the specialized facilities of a health club or Y. If you choose this program, I recommend that you seek instruction in the proper technique and use of the equipment from a qualified personal trainer or health club professional.

Both Fit over Forty Strength Training Programs offer three color-coded program levels to enable you to begin at your current fitness level. Program I includes all the steps you need to achieve and maintain adequate strength and endurance. Since appropriate instruction is recommended, Program II provides only an exercise regimen for each fitness level and a very brief description of each exercise. At the end of each twelve-week program you can maintain that level or retest yourself and move to the next appropriate training level.

STRENGTH TRAINING GUIDELINES

Before we actually discuss specific strength training regimens, I want to give you some background, definitions, and guidelines for performing the exercises that will make your workouts simpler and safer. Then we'll look at some options for scheduling your workouts.

Exercise selection

It's important that your strength training program incorporate exercises that strengthen all of the body's major muscle groups. There are ten major muscle groups in the body: front of the thigh (quadriceps), rear thigh (hamstrings), lower back (erector spinatus), abdominal, chest (pectorals), upper back (rhomboids and trapezius), biceps, shoulders (deltoids), triceps, and neck. The strength training regimens in this book are designed to exercise all these muscle groups. They are also designed to start at your current level of strength and endurance as indicated on your Personal Fitness Profile.

Warm-up and cooldown

Proper warm-up and cooldown are essential to safe and effective strength training. Stretching should be part of both warm-up and cooldown. In Chapter 11, I provide you with a good overall stretching program to use before and after strength training. In addition, warm-up and cooldown should consist of some light exercises for three to five minutes. Alternatively, many people combine their aerobic exercise with strength training, performing the aerobic exercise program first as a warm-up to the strength training session.

Intensity

The best way to maximize the benefit from your strength training program, particularly during the first six months when your greatest strength gains will occur, is to choose an intensity for each exercise that will cause near muscle fatigue by the end of each exercise set. By near muscle fatigue I mean working to the point where you can barely lift the resistance or weight. (For clarity, you should remember that at the first two levels of Program I the weight you are lifting is a portion of your body weight.) The gradual increase in repetitions and/or weight in both programs is designed to provide the proper level of intensity without overworking.

Progression

There are many different methods for determining exercise progression. The one I prefer when using barbells or machines, since it is safe yet highly effective, is called a double progression system. Using this system, you advance by alternatively increasing the weight and number of repetitions. If you are following a barbell or exercise machine routine, you might start with eight repetitions of twenty pounds. You would stay with twenty pounds until you felt comfortable with twelve repetitions. Your next adjustment would be to increase the weight to twenty-one or twenty-two pounds and drop back to eight repetitions. When you are doing calisthenics, as in Program I, your options are a bit more limited. In this instance, initial progression is through an increased number of repetitions. This double progression system kicks in once you add light weights to calisthenic exercise.

The key concept to remember about progression is not to advance repetitions or weight too quickly. In my experience, this is the most common mistake people make. Normally your strength will increase at 2 to 5 percent a week with a well-structured strength training program. This should also be the pace at which you increase resistance, repetitions, or weights. Unfortunately most people want to progress too rapidly. They may be performing a biceps curl at fifteen pounds and a week later add five pounds of resistance. That's a whopping 33 percent increase and an invitation to an injury. Even three pounds represents a 20 percent increase—still too much. A one-pound increase would be about right.

Exercise speed

The key concept related to the speed of strength training exercises is that all the movements should be performed in a slow fashion with controlled movements. This allows the muscles to develop maximum tension and receive the most benefit. In addition, slow, controlled movements minimize the risk of injury that can be caused by rapid, jerky, or out-of-control motions.

Exercise range

Make sure that you perform the strength training exercise through the full range of motion for the muscle. This is essential in order to strengthen the muscle through the entire range that it moves. It's also important so that you retain or increase flexibility. There are certain portions of the range of motion at which each muscle is at its peak strength. If you find that you can move your body (or body part), the weight, or resistance only through this abbreviated range, it means you are progressing too rapidly (too many reps) or are trying to lift too much weight.

Exercise frequency

The optimum frequency for strength training exercises is two to three times a week with a minimum of one day off between sessions. The day off is of critical importance because it allows the muscle to recover from the previous session and maximizes strength gain. Since I enjoy cardiovascular fitness exercise for both health and stress reduction benefits, I find it easiest to perform my strength training after my cardiovascular exercise sessions. I do cardiovascular exercises daily but reserve my strength training to two or three times a week. The Fit over Forty Strength Training Programs are designed for three days a week. But if you want shorter sessions, you can perform the upper body and lower body regimens on alternate days for a six-day schedule.

Breathing

It's important not to hold your breath during strength training exercises since this can result in dangerous temporary increases of blood pressure. Try to breathe continuously during strength training exercise. Most people find that it is most comfortable to breathe in when they're picking up a weight and out when they're putting it down.

Safety

Safety is of critical importance whenever you're strength training, but it's of particular concern as you start your program. If you have any significant medical problem, you should always check with your physician. In addition, proper exercise selection, progression, and good form are keys to injury prevention. I recommend that you seek instruction from a qualified personal trainer, athletic trainer, or health club professional when you get started. Such an individual will not only teach you proper technique and form but also help you select equipment and develop a routine.

Clothing and equipment

For Program I you need comfortable clothing that doesn't get in your way and comfortable athletic shoes; walking shoes, tennis shoes, cross trainers, and running shoes are all fine. Equipment needs are equally simple: (1) a sturdy chair or coffee table, (2) a carpeted floor, exercise mat, or heavy towel, a (dining room/kitchen) table. When (and if) you choose to add weights, you need a selection of handheld dumbbells (one, two, three, four, and five pounds) and ankle weights (weight-adjustable up to ten pounds per ankle). These are available at many sporting goods and fitness stores as well as at hospital supply stores. If you plan to train with free weights or machines, don't rush out and buy them; sign up for proper instruction and a test time at a health club or Y. Failure to follow this advice could result in, at best, a room cluttered with unused equipment, or, at worst, a dangerous injury.

Diet

There is tremendous misinformation about diet and strength training. On the one hand, there are all the various pills and potions that claim to help you improve your muscle tone and build strength. There's not a shred of evidence that any of these work, and they should be avoided. On the other hand, there's a lot of well-meaning but incorrect advice about changing the components of your diet (for example, advice to eat more protein when strength training) to help improve your strength. Once again, there's no evidence to support this concept.

The best diet advice for people who are strength training is to follow the principles of sound human nutrition. I'll be discussing these principles in much greater detail in Chapter 12.

Special medical considerations

In addition to my general advice to check with your physician if you have any concerns about the safety or appropriateness of strength training in your particular circumstances, there are a few specific medical conditions in which strength training is either relatively or absolutely contraindicated. Of course, if you have any significant orthopedic injury or chronic problems with a joint or your back, you'll need to check with your physician and possibly a physical therapist to modify strength training procedures to work for you. Individuals with hypertension should generally not strength train since blood pressure may rise during strength training. If you have hypertension but your blood pressure is well controlled, you may be able to use high repetition, very low weight strength training for muscle toning. Individuals with underlying heart disease need to approach strength training with caution.

If you have any of these conditions, my advice again is to check with your personal physician prior to starting on a strength training regimen.

SCHEDULING YOUR STRENGTH TRAINING SESSIONS

Here are three options for arranging your strength training sessions to fit your goals and schedule:

Three times weekly
1. Do upper and lower body on the same day.
2. In Program I, always complete each exercise A for both upper and lower body before moving on to exercise B for both upper and lower body and so on. Start with squats to begin. In Program II, follow the order given on page 184.
3. Allow at least one day's rest between days (i.e., Monday, Wednesday, Friday or Tuesday, Thursday, Saturday).
4. Warm up and stretch before and after working out.

Six times weekly
This schedule is good for people with small amounts of time available.
1. Do upper and lower body on alternate days (i.e., Monday: upper; Tuesday: lower, etc.).
2. Rest on the day following your third consecutive day of working out (day four); then pick up alternating routine.

Four times weekly
This optional schedule is designed for individuals involved in seasonal sports activities, aerobic workouts, or those who are very active on the weekend.
1. Complete the upper body regimen on Mondays and Thursdays and the lower body regimen on Tuesdays and Fridays.
2. Take Wednesdays off.
3. Take the weekend off.

DETERMINING THE CORRECT STRENGTH TRAINING PROGRAM FOR YOU

To determine the proper program level at which you should start, check your Personal Fitness Profile to see in which category your results on the strength tests placed you: below average, average, or above average. If you scored in different categories for upper and lower body strength, choose the lower category as your starting point for your program for both upper and lower body strength training. Then turn to either Program I, which begins below, or Program II, which begins on page 184. Each program lists the exercises you should perform and gives you a color-coded program chart appropriate for your strength level:

Below average: Blue Program

Average: Yellow Program

Above average: Red Program

Note: If you scored above average but are just beginning a strength program, try Week One of the Red Program, but if it is too difficult, back up and try the Yellow Program.

Each program outlines week by week the number of sets and repetitions in each set you should perform for each exercise. A description of how to perform each exercise then follows.

FIT OVER FORTY STRENGTH TRAINING PROGRAM I

The exercises

Upper Body Regimen

A. Good morning exercise

B. Push-ups/modified push-ups

C. Biceps curls

D. Shoulder raises

E. Triceps dips

F. Abdominal crunches

Lower Body Regimen

A. Squats

B. Knee extension

C. Lunges

D. Hip abduction

E. Hip extension

F. Calf raises

Blue program

Warm up and cool down before each session using the stretching exercises in the next chapter and three to five minutes of light exercise (stationary cycling, walking, jogging). Perform all the exercises in order at all sessions for the indicated sets and repetitions (reps). A set is a group of repetitions. Rest no less than fifteen seconds and no more than a minute and a half between sets. Rest only two to three minutes between exercises.

Week 1:	1 set of 10 reps		
Week 2:	1 set of 11 reps		
Week 3:	1 set of 12 reps		
Week 4:	1 set/10 reps	plus	1 set/3 reps
Week 5:	1 set/10 reps	plus	1 set/4 reps
Week 6:	1 set/10 reps	plus	1 set/5 reps
Week 7:	1 set/10 reps	plus	1 set/6 reps
Week 8:	1 set/10 reps	plus	1 set/7 reps
Week 9:	1 set/10 reps	plus	1 set/8 reps
Week 10:	1 set/10 reps	plus	1 set/9 reps
Week 11:	1 set/10 reps	plus	1 set/10 reps
Week 12:	1 set/11 reps	plus	1 set/10 reps

At the end of twelve weeks, maintain at this level or retest yourself and move on to the Yellow Program.

Yellow program

Warm up and cool down before each session using the stretching exercises in the next chapter and three to five minutes of light exercise (stationary cycling, walking, jogging). Perform all the exercises in order at all sessions for the indicated sets and repetitions (reps). A set is a group of repetitions. Rest no less than fifteen seconds and no more than a minute and a half between sets. Rest only two to three minutes between exercises.

Week 1:	2 sets of 10 reps		
Week 2:	2 sets of 11 reps		
Week 3:	2 sets of 12 reps		
Week 4:	2 sets/10 reps	plus	1 set/5 reps
Week 5:	2 sets/10 reps	plus	1 set/6 reps
Week 6:	2 sets/10 reps	plus	1 set/7 reps
Week 7:	2 sets/10 reps	plus	1 set/8 reps
Week 8:	2 sets/10 reps	plus	1 set/9 reps
Week 9:	2 sets/10 reps	plus	1 set/10 reps
Week 10:	1 set/11 reps	plus	2 sets/10 reps
Week 11:	2 sets/11 reps	plus	1 set/10 reps
Week 12:	3 sets/11 reps		

At the end of twelve weeks, maintain at this level or retest yourself and move on to the Red Program.

Red program

Warm up and cool down before each session using the stretching exercises in the next chapter and three to five minutes of light exercise (stationary cycling, walking, jogging). Perform all the exercises in order at all sessions for the indicated sets and repetitions (reps). A set is a group of repetitions. Add handheld weights or ankle weights to the appropriate exercises (see techniques following) as directed. Rest no less than fifteen seconds and no more than a minute and a half between sets. Rest only two to three minutes between exercises.

Week 1:	3 sets of 10–12 reps		
Week 2:	1 set/10 reps/1 lb weight	plus	2 sets/10 reps/no weight
Week 3:	2 sets/10 reps/1 lb weight	plus	1 set/10 reps/no weight
Week 4:	3 sets/10 reps/1 lb		
Week 5:	1 sets/10 reps/2 lb	plus	2 sets/10 reps/1 lb
Week 6:	2 sets/10 reps/2 lb	plus	1 set/10 reps/1 lb
Week 7:	3 sets/10 reps/2 lb		
Week 8:	1 set/10 reps/3 lb	plus	1 set/10 reps/2 lb
Week 9:	2 sets/10 reps/3 lb	plus	1 set/10 reps/2 lb
Week 10:	3 sets/10 reps/3 lb		
Week 11:	1 set/10 reps/4 lb	plus	2 sets/10 reps/3lb
Week 12:	2 sets/10 reps/4 lb	plus	1 set/10 reps/3 lb

At the end of twelve weeks, maintain at this level or continue adding weights in this progressive pattern until you reach five pounds for the upper body regimen and ten pounds for the lower body regimen.

THE EXERCISES AND HOW TO PERFORM THEM

Exercises for upper body regimen

A. Good Morning Exercise

Stand with feet slightly wider than shoulder-width apart. Keeping your back straight and arms spread wide or on your hips, bend at the hips/waist until your torso is parallel to the floor; then return to starting position. When your torso is parallel to the floor, your head should be up, looking directly in front of you. This exercise should be felt in the lower back and hamstrings.

B. Push-ups/Modified Push-ups

Place hands shoulder-width apart on floor and the balls of your feet on the floor behind you. Keeping your back straight (using your abdominal/back musculature), lower yourself until your waist touches

Program I. A. Good Morning Exercise

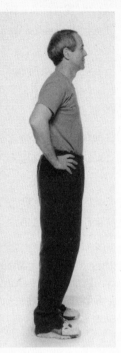
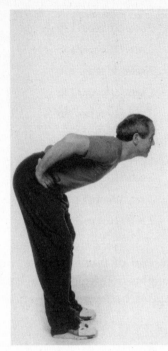

Start   Finish

Program I. B. Push-ups

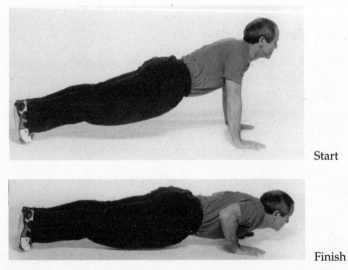

Start

Finish

PROGRAM I. B. Modified Push-ups

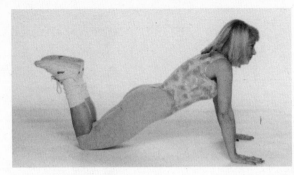

Start

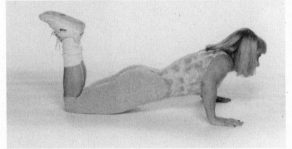

Finish

the floor. Return to starting position. For modified push-ups, stay on your knees rather than your feet throughout entire exercise.

C. Biceps Curls

Start by standing in a comfortable position with your arms at your sides, palms facing forward. Keeping your upper arm straight and close to your body, flex at the elbow until your elbow points directly downward. (In the Red Program this can be done with or without weights.)

D. Shoulder Raises

In a standing position with your arms at your sides and palms facing your legs, raise arms straight out to the side until they are parallel to the floor. Slowly return to starting position. (In the Red Program this can be done with or without weights.)

Program I. C. Biceps Curl

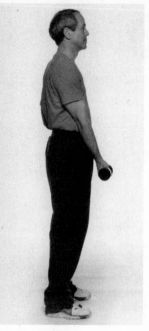
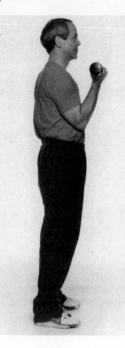

Start   Finish

Program I. D. Shoulder Raises

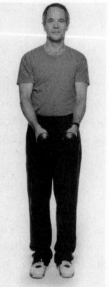

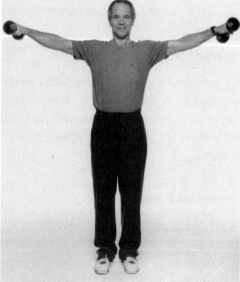

Start   Finish

E. Triceps Dips

Sit on a heavy chair or on the long side of a sturdy coffee table. Place your hands on the edge of the table so your palms are on the top and your knuckles face outward. Place your feet straight out in front of you, and lift your buttocks off the chair/table. Lower yourself toward the floor until your elbows bend to ninety degrees. Return to starting position by using the muscles on the back of your arm.

PROGRAM I. E. Triceps Dips

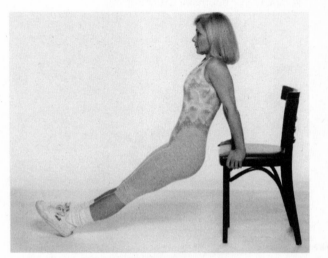

Start

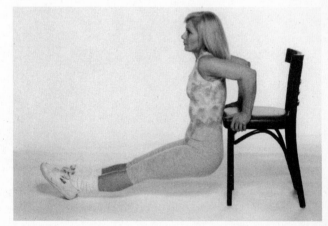

Finish

F. Abdominal Crunches

Lie on a carpeted floor, exercise mat, or thick towel to begin this exercise. Lift your legs off the floor, and bend at the knees so that your legs form a right angle, with your lower legs parallel to the floor. Keeping your lower back on the floor, curl up until your shoulder blades come off the floor, and return to starting position. This exercise should be done very slowly with your hands at your sides or in front of you. It may be helpful to squeeze a ball or towel gently between your knees, as it will better help you to target your abdominal muscles.

PROGRAM I. F. Abdominal Crunches

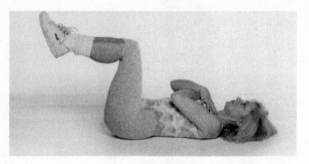

Start

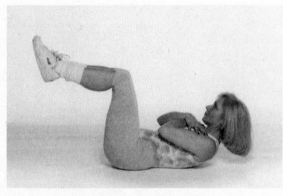

Finish

Exercises for lower body regimen

A. Squats

Stand with your feet shoulder-width apart and pointed slightly outward. Keeping your back straight and head upright, sit slightly backward, and lower yourself to a comfortable position, using your arms to balance yourself. Your knees should always remain directly above your feet and never in front of your toes. Keep your head up during the entire movement, and never look down to check your form (use a mirror if necessary). If your knees are too far forward as you squat, you will need to sit farther backward when beginning the exercise. Your feet should remain flat on the floor at all times, never up on your toes.

PROGRAM I. A. Squats

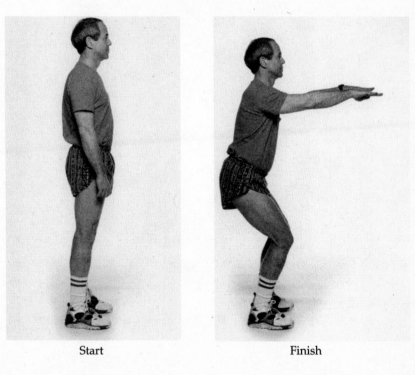

Start   Finish

B. Knee Extension

Get on your hands and knees to begin this exercise. Once in position lift the leg you wish to begin with so that it is straight out behind you. When in this position, flex at the knee until your upper and lower legs touch. Return slowly to starting position. (In the Red Program this exercise can be done with or without ankle weights.)

PROGRAM I. B. Knee Extension

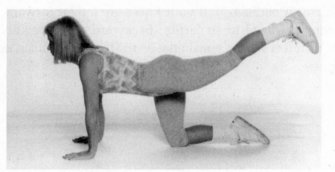

Start

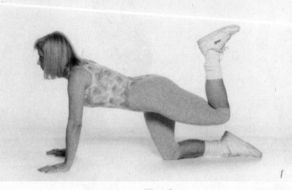

Finish

C. Lunges

Start this exercise standing with your feet about six to eight inches apart. Take a step forward that is slightly larger than usual, and with your back straight, lower your opposite knee slowly to the floor. Push forcefully upward from this position, returning to starting position. Alternate legs for this exercise.

PROGRAM I. C. Lunges

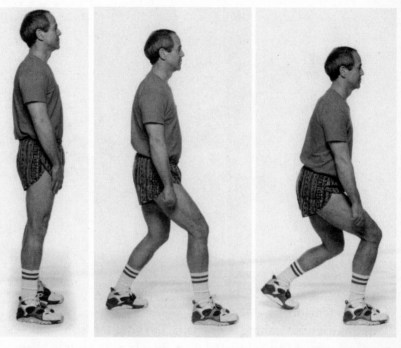

Start   Mid   Finish

D. Hip Abduction

Start this exercise lying on the floor on your side with your feet together. Keeping your body straight, raise your leg out toward your side to a comfortable position; then slowly return to starting position. Use the floor to help keep your balance while leg is in the air. (In the Red Program this exercise can be done with or without ankle weights.)

Program I. D. Hip Abduction

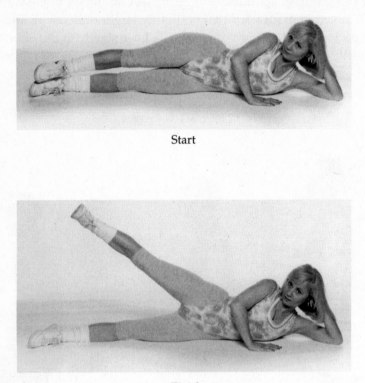

Start

Finish

E. Hip Extension

Start this exercise leaning over a table (on your forearms/elbows) with your legs straight and close together. Slowly raise your leg behind you and away from the table until it is parallel (or almost parallel) to the ground; then slowly return to starting position. (In the Red Program this exercise can be done with or without ankle weights.)

F. Calf Raises

Stand facing a wall or chair with your feet together and knees slightly bent (unlocked). While holding on to the wall for balance rise on your toes (both feet at the same time) and slowly sink back down to the floor.

PROGRAM I. E. Hip Extension

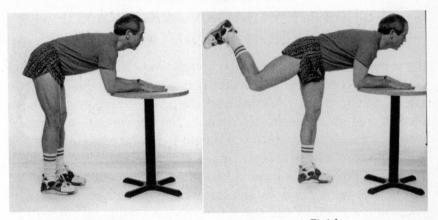

Start   Finish

PROGRAM I. F. Calf Raises

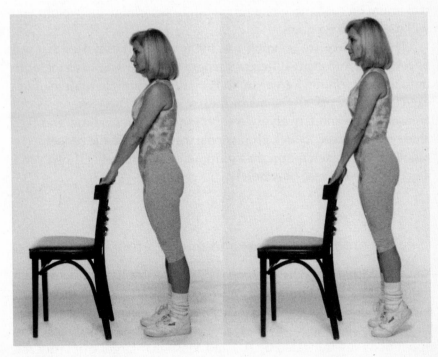

Start   Finish

FIT OVER FORTY
STRENGTH TRAINING PROGRAM II
FOR FREE WEIGHTS AND/OR MACHINES

If you have chosen Program II, the first and most important thing you must do is to get proper instruction. Before you can do these exercises safely and effectively, you must learn the proper techniques and have professional guidance in determining the appropriate amount of weight or resistance at which you should start your program.

Although the Fit over Forty Upper Body and Lower Body Strength Tests have given you a general indication of your strength level, to determine your upper body and lower body strength more precisely, you will need to take additional tests on the equipment you will be using to strength train. Under the supervision of a trained exercise specialist, you will determine the maximum amount of weight you can lift on each piece of equipment. Since this is quite vigorous exercise, it will usually be performed over a two-or three-day period. You will then use a percentage of this figure (typically, approximately 70 percent of your maximum on each piece of equipment) to determine the weight you will use in each program.

Though there are seemingly as many different exercises that can be combined into many different strength training routines as there are individuals training, I give you in Program II a simple routine of ten exercises that work all the major muscle groups. These exercises can be used in the three twelve-week programs—blue, yellow, and red. Since you will need to seek professional instruction on the proper technique for each exercise on the equipment you are using, however, I describe each exercise only briefly.

The order of exercises and muscle group worked

You should perform these exercises in the order listed because the routine starts with the largest muscle groups and works its way to smaller muscles; the sequence also alternates upper body and lower body, a recommended practice. Exercises that target primarily the upper body are indicated by (U) and those that target primarily the abdomen or lower body are indicated by (L).

Bench press: chest (U)

Abdominal crunches or trunk curls: abdomen (L)

Bent-over rows: back (U)

Quadriceps extension: quadriceps (L)

Chest fly: shoulders (U)

Hamstring curls: hamstrings (L)

Biceps curl: biceps (U)

Toe raises with weights on shoulders: calves (L)

Triceps extension: triceps (U)

Wrist roll: forearms (U)

Blue program (starter/below average)

Warm up and cool down before each session using the stretching exercises in the next chapter and three to five minutes of light exercise
(stationary cycling, walking, jogging). Perform all the exercises in order
at all sessions for the indicated sets and repetitions (reps). A set is a
group of repetitions. For all twelve weeks you should use the same
amount of weight or resistance: 70 percent of the maximum weight you
can lift in one repetition for each exercise as determined by the professionally supervised strength tests recommended at the beginning of Program II. Rest no less than fifteen seconds and no more than a minute and
a half between sets. Rest only two to three minutes between exercises.

Week 1:	1 set/10 reps		
Week 2:	1 set/11 reps		
Week 3:	1 set/12 reps		
Week 4:	1 set/10 reps	plus	1 set/3 reps
Week 5:	1 set/10 reps	plus	1 set/4 reps
Weeks 6–12:	Continue adding one rep a week to the second set until you are performing 2 sets of 10 reps each. Then maintain or proceed to the Yellow Program.		

Yellow program (average)

Warm up and cool down before each session using the stretching exercises in the next chapter and three to five minutes of light exercise (stationary cycling, walking, jogging). Perform all the exercises in order at all sessions for the indicated sets and repetitions (reps). A set is a group of repetitions. For all twelve weeks you should use the same amount of weight or resistance: 70 percent of the maximum weight you can lift in one repetition for each exercise as determined by the professionally supervised strength tests recommended at the beginning of Program II. Rest no less than fifteen seconds and no more than a minute and a half between sets. Rest only two to three minutes between exercises.

Week 1:	2 sets/10 reps		
Week 2:	1 set/11 reps	plus	1 set/10 reps
Week 3:	2 sets/11 reps		
Week 4:	1 set/12 reps	plus	1 set/11 reps
Week 5:	2 sets/12 reps		
Week 6:	2 sets/10 reps	plus	1 set/5 reps
Week 7:	2 sets/10 reps	plus	1 set/6 reps
Weeks 8–12:	Continue adding one rep a week to the third set until you are performing 3 sets of 10 reps each. Then maintain or proceed to the Red Program.		

Red program (above Average)

Warm up and cool down before each session using the stretching exercises in the next chapter and three to five minutes of light exercise (stationary cycling, walking, jogging). Perform all the exercises in order at all sessions for the indicated sets and repetitions (reps). A set is a group of repetitions. In the Red Program (unlike the Blue and Yellow Programs) you will be increasing your weight or resistance an average of 3 to 4 percent each week. As you increase weight or resistance, use the double progression method described on page 165. Rest no less than fifteen seconds and no more than a minute and a half between sets. Rest only two to three minutes between exercises.

Week 1:   3 sets/10 reps

Weeks 2–12:   Using the double progression method, add weight or resistance at the rate of 3 to 4 percent per week. Modify your repetitions as appropriate.

A brief description of the exercises in Program II

Bench Press (U)

The bench press, which may be performed with either a barbell or a machine, exercises the chest, front shoulder, and triceps muscles. As you lie on your back on a bench, you lower the weight to mid-chest, then lift it upward until your arms are nearly straight (without locking), and repeat.

Abdominal Crunches or Trunk Curls (L)

The abdominal crunch exercises the abdominal muscles. You perform the exercise lying on the floor with your legs bent at the knees and your arms crossed in front of your upper chest (not behind your head). Keeping your lower back on the floor, slowly curl up until your shoulder blades come off the floor. Return to starting position.

Bent-over Rows (U)

The bent-over row, which is performed with a dumbbell and a bench, exercises the upper back and biceps muscles. You perform the exercise by bending at the waist and placing one hand and one knee on the bench so that your back is parallel to the floor. In your free hand, hold the dumbbell perpendicular to the floor at arm's length, pull it slowly to your chest, then lower it to starting position. If you are using a machine, the upright row is a good substitute.

Quadriceps Extension (L)

The quadriceps extension, which is performed on a machine, exercises the quadriceps muscles, the large muscles in the front of the thighs. To perform the exercise, sit on the seat of your machine with the roller pads over your ankles. Then slowly raise the pads, lifting the weight or resistance, until the quadriceps are fully contracted. Just as slowly return the weight to starting position.

Chest Fly (U)

The chest fly, which may be performed with dumbbells or machines, exercises the chest and front shoulder muscles. To perform the chest fly with dumbbells, you lie on a bench with your feet on the floor, hold the dumbbells above your chest at arm's length, then slowly lower the weight (outward and downward) until the weight is at chest level. Your elbows should be slightly bent. Slowly return your arms and weight to starting position. When using a machine, you produce a similar motion, but you will be sitting up.

Hamstring Curls (L)

Hamstring curls, which are performed on machines, exercise the hamstring muscles, the large muscles in the back of the thighs. Lying facedown on the machine seat or bench, you place the roller pads at the back of your ankles, then slowly bend your knees up, lifting the roller pads until your hamstrings are contracted. Slowly return to starting position.

Biceps Curl (U)

The biceps curl, which may be performed with a barbell, a machine, or dumbbells, exercises the biceps muscles in the front of your upper arms. To perform this exercise, you hold the weight at thigh level with your palms facing out and, keeping your elbows at your sides, slowly lift the weight to shoulder level. Return slowly to starting position.

Toe Raises with Weights on Shoulders (L)

The toe raise, which may be performed with a barbell or machine, exercises the calf muscles in your legs. With the weight on your shoulders and keeping your back and head erect, you slowly lift your heels off the floor, rising on your toes as far as possible, then return slowly to starting position.

Triceps Extension (L)

The triceps extension, which may be performed with dumbbells or on a machine, exercises the triceps muscles in the back of your upper arms. To perform the exercises, you hold the weight in both hands with your arms extended overhead in line with your body. Without moving your elbow from the upright position, you lower the weight behind your neck, then return it to starting position.

Wrist Roll (U)

The wrist roll, which is performed with a bar and weighted rope, exercises the forearm flexor and forearm extensor muscles (your "gripping" muscles). You perform the wrist roll by holding the weighted bar in an overhand grip with your arms extended in front of you. You turn the bar away from you, rolling the weighted rope up on the bar as far as you can, and then turn the bar toward you, rolling the weighted rope off the bar. Using a rubber squeeze doughnut also exercises these muscles well.

WHAT TO EXPECT FROM YOUR
TRAINING REGIMEN

For the first two to four days following your first attempt at the exercise regimen you may be sore. This is usual and is your body's way to let you know it doesn't usually do this sort of exercise. This soreness will not occur after the first couple of training sessions if you are consistent in your workouts. You should wait until you are no longer sore to repeat a regimen (i.e., if your legs are sore until Wednesday from your first lower body workout, you should wait until Thursday, but definitely no later than Friday, to repeat it). If you take a long time off (a week or more) once you have been consistently completing your program, you may get sore when you begin again (although this soreness won't be as intense as when you first began).

This exercise regimen will not immediately change your body; it takes between six and eight weeks of faithfully following the program before any physical changes in your muscle size or shape are possible. You may lose weight from the calories you are expending, but your muscles themselves will not change. During this time your strength and endurance will improve because you are learning how to utilize fully all the muscle you already have. After this initial stage of learning, your body will respond physically through changes in the muscle itself.

This training regimen is designed not to make you gain large amounts of muscle but to make you a healthier individual through the use of a well-rounded exercise regimen. In the process of becoming more physically fit through muscular strength and endurance training you will put on more muscle and may lose some fat. Your weight, however, may not change much or may increase or decrease slightly depending on your body type. Increases in your muscle mass and decreases in your fat mass may balance each other out. Do not measure your success by weight loss; it is often a poor indication of the gains in fitness you have made through muscular strength and endurance training.

The different results produced by this training regime are based on many factors. Some of these are: (1) your current fitness level, (2) the amount of aerobic exercise you are engaged in, and (3) your genetic potential. If you are already a fairly fit person after your initial learning stage, it may be difficult to make large improvements in muscular strength and endurance without a lot of hard work. This, however, does not mean that you should not engage in this type of training regimen, as you will still receive the health benefits that are produced. If you are engaged in a large amount of aerobic activity (running, jogging, rowing, biking, etc.), you also may not experience the same training effects as an individual less aerobically trained. Your genetic potential plays a very important role in the way your body responds to any type of exercise regimen and determines how strong, fast, or large you will become. If you are a naturally thin person, for example, you will certainly experience increased strength and endurance as well as the health benefits, but no change in your size or weight may occur.

GETTING STRONGER

Regular strength training is one of the best *health* decisions you can make at any stage of your life, but particularly over the age of forty. Yet very few of us strength train. On the basis of my experience in medicine and fitness over the past twenty years, I would estimate that less than 5 percent of adults strength train on a regular basis.

Why are so few people involved in strength training? I think it is because most people have a misconception about what strength training is all about. Many people confuse it with body building and envision bulky, dysfunctional muscles built for show rather than function.

Nothing could be further from the truth. Modern strength training builds strong, functional muscles designed to perform at their best throughout our lifetimes. Strength training is one of the great ways we can keep those vital muscles functioning at their best for a lifetime of independent, joyous, healthy living.

CHAPTER 11

FLEXIBILITY: STAYING LOOSE

FLORENCE

Florence hobbled into my office leaning heavily on her cane and plopped down into a chair. I could tell from her grimace when she sat that she was in considerable pain and her scowl indicated that she was also very unhappy.

Florence was a sixty-eight-year-old real estate broker who had been my patient since she suffered a heart attack in her early sixties. Her recovery from the heart attack had been relatively smooth, and after a year's struggle she had managed to kick her lifelong cigarette addiction. She had gained about ten pounds in the year after that (a small price to pay for getting rid of a huge health risk, I reminded her) but still wasn't overweight. She paid attention to what she ate and, in general, took good care of herself. The only negative was that I couldn't get her to exercise. "Too busy," she told me on more than one occasion.

Everything about Florence was usually in overdrive. She moved faster than most people her age, wore a business suit to work each day, and charmed the socks off most people, myself included. It was no wonder that she maintained the most successful real estate practice in central Massachusetts. The last six months, however, had been difficult for her. It had all started with a slip and fall on an icy driveway in December during one of our famous New England ice storms. She had badly twisted her knee and ankle, and since she wouldn't take time to rehabilitate it properly, she struggled for about three months before she could walk normally again. Now she was limping again and very unhappy about it.

"What happened?" I asked.

"I fell again," she lamented, "and this time without any hazard causing it." She went on to explain that she had been showing a house to a client. After looking at the upstairs bedrooms, they had been walking down the stairs to the living room when she had turned around to make one last point. Her foot slightly missed the next step, and she started to fall. Despite an attempt to catch herself on the railing, her feet had slid out from under her, and she went down heavily on her hip and knee. Fortunately she had been near the bottom of the stairs and so had slipped down only two steps. If the carpet had not cushioned her fall somewhat, I would have been visiting her in our intensive care unit with a broken hip.

She had tried to make it through the night, with painkillers, but couldn't sleep. When the morning arrived and the knee and hip were so stiff that she could barely walk, she had called my answering service. I had agreed to fit her in as my first patient at the beginning of clinic hours.

Florence's physical examination revealed a dark purple bruise running from her right buttock halfway down her thigh to her knee and a significant of point tenderness over the hip joint. The hip and knee had such significantly reduced ranges of motion that I had to perform this examination gingerly because of her discomfort. However, even her left hip and knee had significantly smaller range of motion than they should have. Precautionary X rays and an MRI of her hip and knee had revealed no fracture or compromise of the blood supply to the joint, only a deep bruise in the hip area. There was also a minor tear of the lateral cartilage of the right knee that the radiologist and I judged to be old—probably from her fall on the ice the previous December.

I shared with Florence the good news that we had found no fracture and the bad news that the deep hip bruise would put her out of commission for at least a week and make her uncomfortable and slow her down for a few weeks after that. "But the rest of the good news," I said to Florence, "is that I'm finally now going to be able to get you on that walking and stretching program that I've wanted you on all along." Together we planned her rehabilitative program. I scheduled her to see an excellent physical therapist the next day to start passive range-of-motion exercises, followed by a gradual program to increase flexibility in the hip and knee joints and strengthen all the surrounding muscles of the upper leg.

Unfortunately Florence's experience is all too common. Her relatively inactive lifestyle had caused her muscles to become too weak and stiff for the activities of her busy occupation. Since she didn't have a regular program of stretching, her joints had become progressively less flexible. The accidental injury she had incurred when slipping on the ice the previous December had made matters worse and further limited her range of motion. She had compounded the problem by not properly rehabilitating the injured leg. Florence was a broken hip waiting to happen. When she slipped on the stairs, she wasn't strong enough or flexible enough to catch herself, and down she went.

Most people over forty are making the same mistake as Florence. Over age forty subtle changes occur in the tissues of our muscles and joints that make them progressively stiffer and less functional and more injury-prone. Frankly most people are walking around with inadequate levels of flexibility to perform their daily activities safely. They're time bombs waiting for a fall, torn muscle, or even more significant orthopedic injury. Yet in our survey of the fitness habits of people over the age of forty, 47 percent *never* stretch.

It doesn't have to be that way. With a properly designed, simple program of daily stretching exercises you can reverse the decreased mobility that often accompanies aging.

Why don't people pay more attention to maintaining flexibility? I think it's because most don't realize how easy it is to maintain lifelong flexibility and how important it is for overall health and, in their later years, for independent living. Using the simple Fit over Forty Stretching Program presented in this chapter will help you both prepare for your Fit over Forty Walking and Strength Training Programs and improve your flexibility for a lifetime.

Before I describe the program, let's look more closely at how you can benefit from increased flexibility.

BENEFITS OF FLEXIBILITY

Adequate flexibility, which I define as the ability to move your limbs and joints easily the way you need to in order to meet the challenges of daily life, is vital to both an active lifestyle and good health.

Fortunately there's a positive reinforcing cycle between flexibility and activity. Adequate flexibility enables you to maintain an active lifestyle, and an active lifestyle makes an important contribution to maintaining adequate flexibility. These relationships grow stronger the older we become. In one recent study active seventy-year-olds had levels of flexibility more comparable to individuals in their twenties and thirties than inactive people their own age. Staying flexible, therefore, offers several significant benefits. Let's look at a few more of them.

Injury prevention

Since it is closely associated with balance, flexibility is key to injury prevention. In our Advil Fit over Forty Standards research we found a direct relationship between flexibility and balance that became more prominent as people grew older. Longitudinal studies, such as the NIH-funded study in Baltimore, which have followed individuals over a number of decades, have further established this important relationship.

Simply stated, then, a regular program of flexibility exercises is one of the best insurance policies against a debilitating fall, particularly in the later years. Regular stretching exercises also enhance mobility and prevent the type of overextension that leads to muscle pulls or tears or joint damage, such as sprains or cartilage tears. And you're never too old to start such a program. In fact, recent research has shown that regular stretching can significantly improve flexibility in individuals over the age of forty and up into the eighties and nineties.

Improved performance

Enhanced flexibility is also one of the great ways to improve your performance whether in activities around the house or in recreational athletics. As I pointed out in the last chapter, strength training can dramatically improve your distance off the tee or the speed of your tennis serve. So can improved flexibility. You see, in both these activities it's club or racquet speed through the ball that is crucial, and range of motion is critical to the generation of power in both instances.

Slowing the process of aging

There is no question that flexibility declines with age. In part this comes from biochemical changes in muscle and connective tissue. But a much larger contribution comes from inactivity and the cultural expectation that we will become less active as we grow older. While you can't stop the hands on the clock of aging, you sure can slow them down. In fact, if you've never followed a regular stretching routine and use the one I outline in this chapter, you'll find that your flexibility will dramatically improve.

Building strength

Stretching is also a wonderful and vastly underrated technique for building strength. When you relax and stretch one set of muscles, you must contract other muscles (called antagonist muscles) to hold the stretch position. At the most advanced level, some practitioners of yoga are among the strongest people I know simply from holding their stretching positions. Even the mild stretching program I recommend for you in this chapter will result in significant strength benefits within a few months of your starting to do them.

THE FIT OVER FORTY STRETCHING PROGRAM FOR FLEXIBILITY

There are many different stretching exercises available and even some excellent books devoted exclusively to the topic of stretching. The Fit over Forty Stretching Program is a good general stretching program, developed from my laboratory and shown to be safe and effective. You may use this program every day to improve your flexibility whether or not you exercise, and you should also use it as part of your warm-up and cooldown for your walking and strength training programs. In practice, if you have chosen a different cardiovascular fitness activity from walking, you may need to modify the stretching routine slightly to stretch the specific muscles used in your primary fitness activity. A personal trainer can help you here, or consult an excellent book, such as *Stretching* (Shelter Publications) by Bob Anderson, for additional stretches.

As preparation for undertaking the stretching program, we need to consider the important role of stretching in warming up and cooling down, some guidelines for the program, and some tips on how you can use the stretching program to draw on the stress-reducing mind-body connections we've discussed.

FLEXIBILITY, WARMING UP, AND COOLING DOWN

Stretching should always be part of an overall program of warming up and cooling down. It's much easier to stretch muscles and tendons that are already slightly warmed up. Therefore, the procedure I follow, and recommend for you, is to warm up with a little light exercise (perhaps three to four minutes of walking, light pedaling of a stationary cycle, or light jogging) followed by stretching. At the end of a session stretching usually occurs in the middle of the cooldown period.

If you're just stretching on a particular day, the routine is very simple: Warm up; stretch; cool down. You'll be done in ten to fifteen minutes. If you're exercising (either cardiovascular exercise or strength training or both), sandwich the workout between your warm-up and stretching and cooldown and stretching.

One word of caution about the cooldown period: Many people are tempted to skip the cooldown and stretching. Don't make this mistake. Studies in cardiac patients have shown that failure to cool down properly increases the risk of heart rhythm problems. Furthermore, by not cooling down and stretching, you're cheating yourself out of the best time to stretch your muscles, particularly after an exercise session. Skipping the cooldown period and stretching at the end of an exercise session is the most common and serious mistake in flexibility training.

GUIDELINES FOR GETTING THE MOST OUT OF YOUR FLEXIBILITY TRAINING

Over the years I've learned some things, both from my own flexibility training and from observing the hundreds of individuals who come through our exercise programs, that can help make your flexibility training program safer, more enjoyable, and more effective. Here are a few tips.

1. Check with your physician before starting any exercise program. It's particularly important if you have been very sedentary.

2. Incorporate your stretching into your warm-up and cooldown. Incorporate the advice given in the previous section.
3. Stretch slowly, and pay attention to breathing deeply as you do. You should stretch until you feel a slight tugging or pulling sensation. Never stretch to the point of actual pain. Also, don't bounce during your stretch. That's called ballistic stretching, and it not only decreases the effectiveness of the stretch but can actually injure the muscle or joint. Hold each stretch for seven to ten seconds. Then gently ease away from it.
4. If you've had an injury, take special precautions. If you've had a major injury to a muscle or joint, ask your physician to arrange an appointment with a physical therapist or athletic trainer. These professionals have special training in designing safe and effective stretching programs for individuals recovering from injuries. If you've had a minor injury, proceed cautiously. Move into and out of each stretch more slowly and never proceed to the point of actual pain.

USING THE MIND-BODY CONNECTIONS OF YOUR FLEXIBILITY PROGRAM

As you know from previous chapters, I'm a firm believer in mind-body interactions and their potential to yield multiple health benefits. In my own fitness regimen I use the warm-up and cooldown and stretching periods as times when I'm particularly conscious of working on mind-body interactions (and reaping the relaxing, stress-reducing benefits of this focus).

During my warm-up and stretching I start to listen to my breathing and feel the state of my body and mind. I begin to fall into the rhythm of the exercise and take an inventory of my body and mind. My mind begins to float, and I begin to visualize the pleasure I anticipate from the workout. By the time I'm ready to start the exercise session, I am already deeply into the mind-body aspects of it and am very relaxed. A similar process occurs at cooldown and stretching except during this period I'm slowly coming out of the mind-body sphere and experiencing and cataloging what I've accomplished.

One trick that my friend Ruth Stricker taught me about mind-body interactions and how to evoke them is the Chinese concept of soft eyes. According to Ruth, we tend to glare and see things with hard eyes.

Trying to see things softly and bring a soft expression to your eyes is a wonderful entrée into mind-body consciousness. I often think "soft eyes" when I'm warming up or cooling down, and the concept usually carries over into my workout.

HOW TO CONDUCT THE FIT OVER FORTY STRETCHING PROGRAM

The stretching program is divided into upper and lower body exercises, described and illustrated below. Each exercise targets a specific major muscle group. Again, it is important to concentrate on what you are doing and to listen to what your body is telling you. Perform the exercises in the order given.

Before You Start: Be sure to begin with a light five- to ten-minute warm-up to increase circulation, warm up muscles, and generally prepare the body for the exercises. The warm-up can be light calisthenics, a brisk walk, jogging in place, or cycling.

During the Exercise: It is essential to progress slowly and to be consistent with your program. Begin the program by holding each position for ten seconds. As you increase your flexibility and range of motion, hold the position for fifteen to twenty seconds. It is not necessary to perform each exercise for more than twenty seconds.

After You Finish Stretching: End your stretching exercise program with a cooldown, repeating the same warm-up activities, but at a slower pace, for an additional five to ten minutes.

THE STRETCHING EXERCISES

Upper body program

Full Body Stretch

Lying supine, extend your arms straight over your head and your legs straight out (pointing your toes) in the opposite direction. Reach; extend and hold for ten seconds; relax. Repeat two or three times.

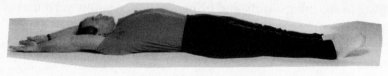

FIGURE 11.1. Full Body Stretch

Full Upper Body Stretch

Sitting, with legs bent underneath you, reach forward with both arms extended forward while pressing your palms to the floor. This can also be performed one arm at a time. Reach for ten seconds; then relax. Repeat two or three times.

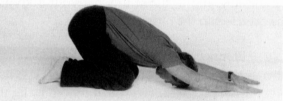

FIGURE 11.2. Full Upper Body Stretch

Shoulders and Outer Portions of Arms and Ribs

While sitting cross-legged or standing upright, extend your arms over your head, pull your palms together (as shown), and stretch your arms upward and slightly backward (behind your head). Hold for ten seconds; then relax. Repeat two or three times.

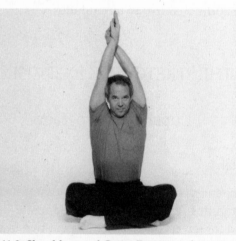

FIGURE 11.3. Shoulders and Outer Portions of Arms and Ribs

Shoulders and Middle Back

While sitting or standing, draw your arm across your chest toward the opposite shoulder by pushing in at your elbow. Perform this on both the left and right sides. Hold each stretch for ten seconds, and then relax. Repeat two or three times with each arm.

Side Stretch

While standing with knees slightly bent, gently pull your elbow up behind your head. In the same motion, bend from the hips to the same side. Hold for ten seconds; then relax. Repeat two or three times on each side.

Shoulder and Neck Stretch

Leaning your head toward your right shoulder, pull your right arm down across behind your back with your left hand. Perform this exercise on both sides, holding each stretch for ten seconds and then relaxing. Repeat two or three times on each side.

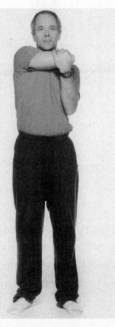

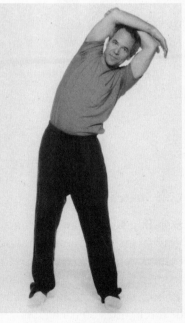

FIGURE 11.4. Shoulders and Middle Back   FIGURE 11.5. Side Stretch

Arms, Shoulders, and Chest

Extend your arms back behind your back, and clasp hands together. Then slowly pull your interlocked fingers upward. Hold for ten seconds; then relax. Repeat two or three times.

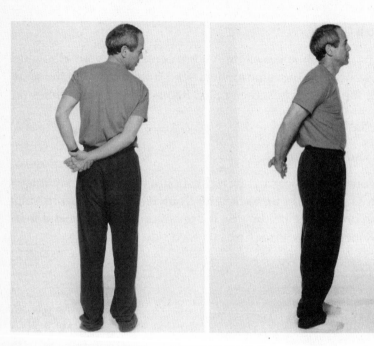

FIGURE 11.6. Shoulder and
Neck Stretch

FIGURE 11.7. Arms, Shoulders,
and Chest

Lower body program

Calf Stretch

Standing slightly away from a wall or a steady support, lean on it with your arms. Bend one leg, and keep the other leg slightly bent back behind you. Move your hips forward toward the wall while attempting to keep the heel of the back leg flat on the ground. Perform the stretch on both sides, holding each stretch for ten to thirty seconds. Repeat two or three times on each side.

Groin Stretch

While sitting on the floor with the balls of the feet together (as shown) and the back straight, attempt to push your knees outward and toward the ground. Hold the position for ten seconds; then relax. Repeat two or three times, performing the exercise slowly because very little movement will elicit a stretch.

Hamstring Stretch

While sitting with legs extended outward (slightly bent) and in the straddle position, bend forward at the hips, reach toward one leg, and hold. Then reach toward the middle, and hold; finally reach toward the opposite leg, and hold. Perform this two or three times in each of the three positions slowly and deliberately.

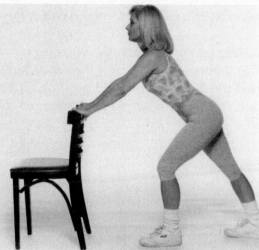

FIGURE 11.8. Calf Stretch

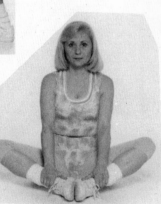

FIGURE 11.9. Groin Stretch

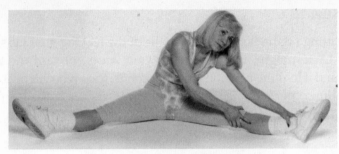

FIGURE 11.10. Hamstring Stretch

Quadriceps (Thigh) Stretch

Stretch 1: Sitting with one leg extended outward and the other leg bent in the hurdler's position (with the foot pointing outward from the body), begin to lean slightly backward. Move slowly and deliberately since this exercise requires little movement to elicit a stretch response. Hold the position for ten seconds; then relax. Perform this two or three times on each side.

Stretch 2: With one knee resting on the floor and the other leg out in front (the knee of the front leg should be directly over the ankle), lower the front of your hip toward the floor slowly. Hold position for ten seconds; then relax. Perform this exercise two or three times on the right and left sides.

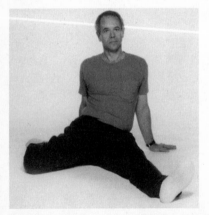

FIGURE 11.11. Quadriceps (Thigh) Stretch 1

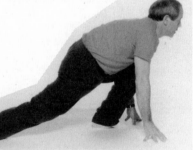

FIGURE 11.12. Quadriceps (Thigh) Stretch 2

Ankle Rotation

While sitting cross-legged, roll one foot in a circle clockwise and counterclockwise. Perform this exercise three or four times in each direction on both ankles.

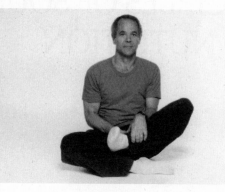

FIGURE 11.13. Ankle Rotation

IMPROVED FLEXIBILITY AND COMPREHENSIVE FITNESS

I view stretching exercises to improve flexibility as the "unknown soldier" of a comprehensive fitness program. Adequate flexibility is crucial to good health, injury prevention, and daily performance. Yet far too few people know about this and act on it.

Adequate flexibility is also crucial to the safe and effective performance of cardiovascular fitness exercises and strength training. Fortunately, flexibility training is linked to these other exercises in a positive reinforcing cycle. Adequate flexibility assures that you can perform cardiovascular fitness exercises and strength training, and both these latter activities result in improved flexibility. Flexibility training is also a wonderful window for stimulating mind-body interactions.

I love telling you about flexibility training. It's simple and pleasurable, takes little time, and results in multiple health and fitness benefits. What could be better than that?

CHAPTER 12

EATING RIGHT: PRINCIPLES OF SOUND NUTRITION

JIM

Jim. Ah, Jim. His problems started around the time he turned forty, or maybe it's more accurate to say that's when he first began to notice them.

Jim had been extremely active throughout his life—first as a high school and college athlete, and subsequently in a variety of sports and recreation activities, including an extensive running and walking program. It was a rare day when he didn't get in either a thirty- to forty-five-minute jog or fitness walk. So far, so good. Jim was living up to many of the principles I've already discussed. But this is a chapter about nutrition, not physical activity. And there, truth be told, Jim wasn't doing a particularly good job.

He traced his problems back to his late thirties, when he began to notice that for the first time in his life, his weight was starting to creep up. At thirty-five he weighed 155 pounds, the same he had weighed during college and an excellent weight for his five-foot-nine-inch frame. Like many others, he had experienced one bout of weight gain during graduate school, but that had quickly melted away with his running program in his late twenties and early thirties. In his late thirties Jim began to notice some subtle changes. He started gaining a little

weight—just a pound or two each year, but despite his program of vigorous physical activity, it stayed on. By the age of forty he weighed 161
pounds, a relatively small change, but it made his suits fit a little too
tightly. Projecting forward, he realized that he was gaining at a rate of
ten pounds a decade. A weight of 171 at age fifty seemed both highly
possible and unappealing. Weighing in at 181 at age sixty would be
downright appalling. As important, Jim began to notice small changes
in his energy level. He felt more sluggish than he wanted to and often
had a period of several hours after lunch when he felt a bit drowsy.

Acting on these observations, Jim made what, in retrospect, was a
brilliant decision. Since he figured that his weight gain and drowsiness
were possibly related to what he ate, he made an appointment to see a
nutritionist. The results of Jim's nutritional evaluation were informative and shocking. The nutritionist put him through a rigorous evaluation, including three-day food records (where he kept track of
everything he ate for three days), followed by computer analysis of the
data, an hour nutritional counseling session, and a body fat analysis.
Here's what was found.

Jim's overall calorie consumption was high at more than three
thousand calories a day. Since his height and baseline weight suggested
that twenty-four hundred calories were appropriate for maintaining a
stable weight, he got away with this potentially disastrous calorie consumption (as so many recreational athletes do) because his daily four-
and-one-half-mile jog or run burned an average of over five hundred
calories, almost, but not quite, bringing him into balance. His food
intake was overshooting his daily calorie use by only one to two hundred calories—not much but, over a period of months and years,
enough to set up the creeping weight gain he had experienced.

The composition of Jim's diet was an even bigger problem. It consisted of 40 percent of his calories from fat, 45 percent from carbohydrates, and 15 percent from protein. The numbers shocked him. Jim
prided himself on being health-conscious and couldn't believe he was
consuming 25 percent more calories from fat than recommended by the
American Heart Association and every other responsible nutritional
authority. A little detective work found the culprits.

Jim started off the day in a reasonable fashion. His daily breakfast
of cereal with low-fat milk or toast with jam often accompanied by a
piece of fruit, a glass of juice, and a cup of coffee might, as we'll see
later in the chapter, be criticized as a little light on calories. But at least

it was a real breakfast, consistently consumed and also low in fat. Lunch was the problem. Jim started off by packing his own lunch—an excellent practice I heartily endorse—and the ingredients were typically well thought out: a tuna fish or turkey sandwich and a piece of fruit. But from there it went downhill. Jim had slipped into the practice of "supplementing" his lunch at work. A quick trip to the vending machines resulted in a couple of cookies, a bag of Doritos, and a can of soda. This "modified" lunch often contained over nine hundred calories, over 50 percent of which were from fat. It was also laden with sugar and caffeine—a combustible combination, causing a sugar explosion followed by an insulin outpouring and subsequent period of low blood sugar. No wonder he was drowsy after lunch and gaining weight! Dinner marked a bit of a comeback to nutritional sanity, although it often contained a few too many calories and, because of the stress of work, was often consumed too late.

The bad news was that Jim's nutritional practices had started to create predictable problems for him—both weight gain and fatigue—and, unless they were turned around, could ultimately lead to significant health problems. The good news was that they were eminently correctable through small changes in his diet. Jim and his nutritionist formed a strategy to get him back on track.

Before I continue, let me make a confession. I pride myself in following my patients' lifestyle practices in great detail, but my detailed knowledge of Jim's nutrition goes beyond what any doctor knows about any patient. The reason for this is simple: I'm talking about myself.

Over the years, like many people, I had drifted into nutritional habits that were unhealthy. It's incredibly easy to do this. In fact, in our culture, packed with high-calorie foods that are laden with fat and sugar, it's actually difficult to avoid falling into nutrition traps. These foods are quick, convenient, and, yes, often incredibly tasty. So we all face challenges on the nutritional front on a daily basis, whether or not we are making healthy choices, such as regular physical activity, in other areas of our lives. In fact, in my experience over the years in caring for hundreds of physically active individuals, I've found these people often have *worse* nutritional habits than less active individuals. I would estimate that less than 10 percent of these active individuals pay as much attention to their nutrition as to their exercise. Instead many use their exercise program, as I did, as a vehicle to control their weight—a big mistake.

Let's return for a moment to my nutritional awakening. Seeing a nutritionist was of course easy for me since my laboratory performs research in this area and I had four full-time nutritionists on my staff. The changes Marcie asked me to make were amazingly simple. We started with the lunch problem. What I liked about the Doritos was the fact that they provided something crunchy with my sandwich. The switch to melba toast was simple. The cookies were superfluous and were discarded. My choice of beverage had been rather unconscious, as it is for many people. Soda was convenient, but what my body was really calling for was the water it contained. The switch to bottled water was also easy (I actually prefer the taste) and immediately eliminated tons of sugar and caffeine from my diet.

The changes I made were so simple and made such an enormous difference in my life that I am almost embarrassed to recount this entire episode. Within a week of committing to these minor alterations in my lunch menu, I could notice significant change. Almost immediately my early-afternoon drowsiness departed and my energy rebounded. No surprise there—I wasn't battling hypoglycemia while trying to digest a high-fat meal! Within two weeks the changes had become routine. Within three months my weight had drifted back to its long-standing 155 pounds—without a single alteration in my lifestyle.

Physician, heal thyself!

NUTRITION AND HEALTH

Somehow as a society we've become blind to the links between sound nutrition and good health. I'm not sure exactly why this is. Perhaps many, as I did, simply drift slowly into unhealthy eating patterns without knowing it. Maybe the pervasive advertising of high-fat, high-calorie, convenient processed foods lulls us into habits that we don't consciously examine. Or confronted by such a clutter of seemingly conflicting information on what constitutes good nutritional practices, we just dismiss the whole confusing business and go on as we always have. Whatever the reason, ignoring the links between sound nutrition and good health is tantamount to playing with fire. The surgeon general's report on nutrition released in the late 1980s draws a startling conclusion: Seven out of ten leading causes of death in the United States have a nutritional or alcohol-related component!

For example, as I'll discuss more fully below, the linkage between heart disease and such nutritional practices as overconsumption of saturated fat and cholesterol is well established. Nutrition also makes a vastly underestimated contribution to cancer since more than half of all cancers have a nutritional component. And when you factor poor nutritional practices—the overconsumption of both fat and calories—into the equation for obesity, you're looking at a public health problem of enormous magnitude. I could go on and on with this list; there's really no condition or disease process in which nutritional practices are irrelevant.

Looking at this evidence, I want to emphasize two key points: First, poor nutritional practices contribute to every major health problem that bedevils us; second, good nutritional patterns—if we understand what they are and adopt them—can play a critical role in enhancing our health, happiness, and quality of life.

CUTTING THROUGH THE CONFUSION ABOUT GOOD NUTRITION

The late president John F. Kennedy was fond of saying, "Knowledge is power," as he urged our nation into the space and computer ages. Who could deny the importance of knowledge as the basis for informed decisions? Yet in the area of nutrition we have almost driven this concept beyond a manageable level. If nutritional knowledge is power, I've come to believe that too much knowledge, particularly if not filtered through critical analysis, can lead to chaos and confusion.

As the medical editor of the Television Food Network I've had the responsibility of combing the nutritional literature over the past few years and trying to help people put studies in perspective. This experience has left me with one overriding conclusion: We accept many ideas, theories, and studies in the area of nutrition much too uncritically. I've seen studies with as few as ten or twenty individuals reported in the media as though they were major scientific breakthroughs. I've seen authors come through our station promoting books with "new" nutritional concepts that are as *ridiculous* as they are novel.

While research in the last few years has produced some phenomenally important new information in the area of nutrition, there is also a good deal of garbage that passes for "expert" opinion. While the topic of nutrition is truly vast, I don't think it has to be confusing. There are concepts and practices that have stood the test of time and are recognized by every leading legitimate nutritional authority in our country.

These practices, if put into place in all our diets, could have tremendous immediate and long-term health benefits for all of us.

That's what this chapter is about: cutting through the nutritional clutter that's out there and giving you some practical advice to put into practice in your life immediately. Since the basic information you need is actually very simple—and there's no one right way to carry it out—this chapter features practical information and tips that you can adapt to your needs. If your Personal Fitness Profile indicated that you also need to lose weight, the next chapter contains the Fit over Forty Eating Plan for Weight Management, which is based on the principles of nutrition presented in this chapter.

HEALTHY PLEASURES

I'm not a food cop. Most of the writing I've seen about good nutritional practices suffers from a common flaw: It lectures about bad habits and somehow makes healthy eating seem, well, unappetizing. What these writers fail to recognize is that food is far more than just nutrition. It's joy and celebration and sharing. It's multicolored, tactile, and sensual. It's one of the ways we both give and get love. It's one of life's great pleasures and one of the ways we connect with one another and the earth. I love food. I love to eat, cook, and share food. And yes, I care deeply about food and health, but first and foremost, food is a healthy pleasure.

Before I went to medical school, I was an avid amateur chef—and remain so to this day. I've prepared many of the recipes from Julia Child's two-volume masterpiece on French cooking (*Mastering the Art of French Cooking*) and make most of James Beard's bread recipes. I cooked in a French restaurant for six months prior to entering medical school. My wife and I derive intense pleasure from preparing and eating fine food, and the kitchens in our houses are a focal point. While I'm always on the lookout for ways to cut fat from recipes, I believe the pleasure of cooking and preparing food has been vastly underrated as health-promoting behavior. Lest I lose my union card in the union of cardiologists, I want to hasten to point out that we cook classic French food only occasionally. A typical meal for us is broiled fresh fish (we do live in Boston after all), pasta or potato, and fresh vegetables accompanied by a shared bottle of wine.

I recount these gastronomic facts as background for one reason: I firmly believe that sound nutrition is a key to good health. I also believe that we eat for pleasure, good company, celebration, and joy, and these are essential to good health as well. Pleasure and good nutrition are not incompatible. I think they're inseparable. People who spend their lives at war with food—whether it's eating too much and never tasting it or fearing it and never enjoying it—are not only missing one of life's greatest pleasures but also risking their health.

PRINCIPLES OF
SOUND NUTRITION

A few years ago a number of the major health and nutrition organizations in the United States came together to try to articulate some guidelines for our diet. The guidelines they generated are extremely well done and easy to follow. Yet getting the message out has proved a greater challenge. Few people have ever heard of the guidelines, let alone put them into practice.

In my mission to boil nutrition down into some bite-size, easily digestible nuggets, I'm going to take two steps. In this section I'm going first to list and then to interpret the nine principles that form the American Heart Association and American Dietetic Association guidelines for healthy eating. In the next section I'll distill the brew even further into the three nutritional practices I believe are the keys to good health. Then it's your job to begin to apply these principles to your own practices.

THE AHA/ADA DIETARY
GUIDELINES

1. Limit saturated fat intake to less than 10 percent of fat calories.
2. Limit total fat intake to less than 30 percent of total calories.
3. Cholesterol intake should be limited to less than 100 mg per thousand calories and not more than a total of 300 mg a day.
4. Increase the amount of carbohydrate in the diet to 50 to 55 percent of the total calories or more. Emphasize complex carbohydrates.
5. Limit sodium intake to no more than 1 gram per thousand calories and not more than a total of 3 grams a day.
6. Protein should comprise approximately 15 percent of the total calories.
7. If you consume alcoholic beverages, do not exceed 1 to 1.5 ounces of alcohol a day (approximately one shot of distilled spirits or two glasses of wine or two beers).

8. Do not consume more calories than are required to maintain your best body weight.
9. Consume a variety of food.

Let's look at each of these principles in a little more detail.

Lower the fat in your diet

This objective combines the first two AHA/ADA principles. Lowering the fat in our diet, particularly the saturated fat, which typically, although not always, comes from animal sources, is of critical importance to our health. In fact, the surgeon general's report cited earlier lists the overconsumption of fat as the number one nutritional problem facing Americans today. The reasons for this stern warning are simple. Extra fat consumption in the diet leads to two significant health problems: obesity and elevated cholesterol. A diet high in fat has also been linked to heart disease, colon cancer, and diabetes.

The scorecard on fat consumption in our country is somewhat mixed. On the good-news side, the level of fat consumption has declined over the past ten years. In the past decade the percentage of calories we consume from fat has declined from 40 percent of total calories to 34 percent. On the bad-news side, this is still far too much fat. Furthermore, in terms of weight control, as we'll see later, simply lowering fat is not enough; calories also count.

When we talk about lowering saturated fats, we are talking about lowering one type of fat. There are essentially three types of fat: saturated, monounsaturated, and polyunsaturated. Animal fats are typically saturated and are generally solid at room temperature. Plant and vegetable fats are typically monounsaturated or polyunsaturated and are generally liquid at room temperature, although there are exceptions to this rule, such as palm oil, coconut oil, and chocolate, all of which are loaded with saturated fat. Saturated fats tend to raise blood cholesterol and, in general, should be limited to no more than 10 percent of total calories. Substituting saturated fat with either monounsaturated or polyunsaturated fats lowers cholesterol; thus the less saturated fats are better choices.

Here are common fat sources that you can use as a guide as you work to lower saturated fats in your diet:

Saturated Fats	Monounsaturated Fats	Polyunsaturated Fats
Animal Sources	*Animal Sources*	*Animal Sources (of omega-3 fatty acids)*
Cheese	Chicken	Fish
Butter	Fish	
Milk		*Plant Sources*
Meat	*Plant Sources*	Walnuts
Eggs	Vegetable oil	Filberts
Lard	Pecans	Soft margarine
	Olive oil	Almonds
Plant Sources	Canola oil	Mayonnaise
Coconut oil	Stick margarine	Soybean oil
Palm oil	Peanut oil	Corn oil
Palm Kernel oil	Peanut butter	Sunflower oil
Cocoa butter	Cottonseed oil	Safflower oil
(chocolates)	Avocados	Sesame oil

Among these categories, monounsaturated fats seem to be particularly beneficial. In fact, I believe, as do many cardiologists, that the high level of monounsaturated fats (largely from olive oil) in the diets of Mediterranean countries makes a major contribution to the strikingly low incidence of heart disease in this region. Over the past few years my wife and I have turned almost exclusively to olive oil for our source of fat in our diet. The monounsaturated fats seem to have the dual advantage of raising HDL (the good cholesterol) without raising total cholesterol. The American Diabetes Association has also recognized the value of monounsaturated fats in the diet and recommended increased consumption of them for most diabetics. The one downside: Like any fat, they contain a lot of calories.

Lower your cholesterol consumption and control blood cholesterol

We've heard a lot about lowering our blood cholesterol levels over the past decade. Unfortunately there has been a swing toward revisionism over the past few years with even some otherwise well-informed physicians making the misguided argument that the risk of an elevated blood cholesterol level has been overstated.

Let me state my view on this clearly. Every adult should know his or her blood cholesterol level, which is determined from a simple blood test, and strive to keep it below 200 mg/dl. Once your blood cholesterol level rises above 200 mg/dl, the risks of heart disease start rising rapidly. The first line of therapy for elevated cholesterol is dietary intervention to lower both saturated fat and cholesterol consumption.

There are two major sources of cholesterol in our body; we manufacture some and consume the rest. It is the latter area to which we need to pay more attention. The American Heart Association recommends that the average adult consume no more than 300 mg of cholesterol a day. Yet the average adult in our society consumes over 400 mg of cholesterol a day—almost 33 percent too much.

Cholesterol is a naturally occurring waxy substance that is found only in animal tissue. It is present particularly in red meat, eggs, and dairy products. It makes up a vital element of animal cell membranes and also plays a key role in the production of many of the body's hormones. A certain amount of cholesterol is therefore vital to life itself. It is only when it gets too high that it causes problems. Cholesterol is carried around in the bloodstream attached to structures called lipoproteins. When the cholesterol level gets too high, the excess can be deposited on the inside of arterial walls, causing them to narrow. The end result can be coronary heart disease and angina, or a heart attack.

Within the class of lipoproteins that are involved in the transport of cholesterol, some are more dangerous than others. High levels of the low density lipoproteins (LDL) and very low density lipoprotein (VLDL) are associated with increased risk of heart disease while the high density lipoprotein (HDL) actually confers some protective effects. The best way to raise HDL? You guessed it: regular exercise!

Increase the amount of carbohydrate in the diet to 50 to 55 percent of total calories

There's almost nothing bad to say about carbohydrates—particularly the complex carbohydrates found in fruits, vegetables, and grains. Other great sources of carbohydrates are breads, cereals, rice, and pasta.

The truth is that we don't eat enough of these foods—but be careful about the sauces. Sometimes people eat pasta in an Italian restaurant thinking they're eating a healthy meal, and they are—unless it's drenched in a high-fat Alfredo sauce or loaded with sausage!

Limit sodium intake

As a society we consume far too much sodium, largely in the form of sodium chloride, common table salt. The average adult consumes six to eight grams of salt a day—more than twice the three-gram limit recommended by the American Heart Association. The major reason to avoid salt is its association with high blood pressure. Certainly individuals with histories of high blood pressure ought to minimize salt in their diets. When I convince my patients with hypertension to limit salt strictly and to control their weight, many are able to manage their blood pressure without medication.

Here are a few easy ways to cut down on salt:

1. Cut down on fast and processed foods; they are usually loaded with salt.
2. Never salt your food before tasting it.
3. Take the salt shaker off the table. If you have to stand up to get it, you will at least think twice about using it.

Limit your protein intake to 15 percent of total calories

The average American diet contains far too much protein, yet for years I've been hearing so-called fitness experts advocate increased protein consumption for building muscle. There isn't a shred of evidence, however, that increased protein consumption above a normal healthy, varied diet helps build muscle, and at some level much increased protein in the diet may actually become dangerous to your kidneys.

To put in perspective how far the average person's diet exceeds needed protein, let me tell you that if you have a chicken sandwich and an eight-ounce glass of milk for lunch, you've fulfilled your recommended daily allowance for protein.

If you still think you need to load up on protein before strenuous activity—like playing a big game, running a marathon, or digging the garden—think again. What do the pros now eat? High-carbohydrate meals. Thankfully the pregame ritual of eating steaks and other meat-laden meals has been relegated to the junk heap of food myths, where it belongs. Since most of the calories in such a meal are fat, all the meal does is slow you down during competition as your body tries valiantly to digest it.

If you consume alcohol, do so in moderation

Alcohol consumption is a complex issue. Now I'm never going to suggest to any patient who doesn't consume alcohol that he or she start. And I certainly don't advocate or condone excessive alcohol consumption. Yet in the past few years several studies have shown that the moderate consumption of alcohol significantly reduces the risk of heart disease and heart attack.

Alcohol seems to confer these benefits through two mechanisms. First, it raises the blood level of HDL cholesterol, and increased levels are associated with decreased risk of heart disease. Second, some forms of alcoholic beverages also impede blood clotting, and blood clotting is part of the process of heart attacks. This latter benefit seems unique to red wine and is thought to come from flavinoids, substances found particularly in the skins of grapes that are left in the process of wine-making much longer in red wine than in white. Incidentally, red grape juice has the same effect, but you have to drink twice as much.

How much is "moderate" alcohol consumption? One shot of distilled spirits, two glasses of wine, or two beers. Levels of alcohol consumption above this carry a variety of unacceptable risks, such as liver disease, certain cancers of the gastrointestinal tract, and accidents of all kinds—most prominently motor vehicle accidents.

Don't take in more calories than required to maintain your best body weight

Weight management and the health consequences of obesity are of such profound importance that I've devoted the next chapter to them. Let me just state for now that calories do count! For a long time we used to think that if we could lower fat consumption in our country, weights would automatically come tumbling down. I've been a longtime advocate of lowering fat consumption for all the reasons we've already discussed. However, our experience over the past decade has clearly taught us that calories count as well.

During a time when fat consumption has fallen dramatically, calorie consumption has actually increased, and the incidence of obesity has exploded. The trouble is we've replaced high-fat products with equally high-calorie processed foods loaded with simple sugars. This latter point was driven home to me at the Television Food Network one night when we received a fervid press release announcing that SnackWell's chocolate cookies had surpassed Oreos as the number one cookie in America, ending a decade of Oreo dominance. SnackWell's claim to fame: no fat. The difference in calories between SnackWell's and Oreos—almost none! Calories count.

Consume a variety of foods

We all heard when we were growing up that the keys to good nutrition were balance, variety, and moderation. Well, guess what? That advice turns out to be true, only now we have a better understanding of what these words mean and a powerful tool to help us sort through the nutritional maze. It's called the Food Guide Pyramid.

The Food Guide Pyramid was developed by the U.S. Department of Agriculture and the Department of Health and Human Services. It goes beyond and replaces the Four Food Groups that we all grew up on. I believe that the Food Guide Pyramid offers an excellent tool to guide people to eat a healthy diet based on the principles of balance, variety, and moderation. It even goes one step beyond. It puts the guidelines for healthy eating that we've already discussed into action by recommending the amounts of each type of food we should consume. Let's take a brief look at the Food Guide Pyramid.

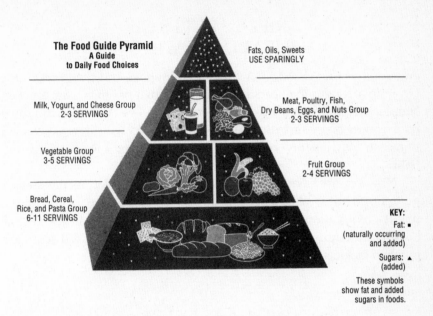

The Food Guide Pyramid
A Guide
to Daily Food Choices

Fats, Oils, Sweets
USE SPARINGLY

Milk, Yogurt, and Cheese Group
2-3 SERVINGS

Meat, Poultry, Fish,
Dry Beans, Eggs, and Nuts Group
2-3 SERVINGS

Vegetable Group
3-5 SERVINGS

Fruit Group
2-4 SERVINGS

Bread, Cereal,
Rice, and Pasta Group
6-11 SERVINGS

KEY:
Fat: ■
(naturally occurring
and added)
Sugars: ▲
(added)
These symbols
show fat and added
sugars in foods.

The Food Guide Pyramid provides a pictorial guide to the principles of sound nutrition. As you can see, the fats, oils, and sweets (loaded with simple sugars) are positioned in the small apex of the pyramid, indicating that they should be used sparingly. The fruits and vegetables and other carbohydrate-rich foods form the bottom two layers of the pyramid, indicating that they should form the solid basis of a healthy diet.

I discuss the Food Guide Pyramid with all my patients and recommend it as an excellent basis for sound nutrition. There are also fine pamphlets available from the U.S. Department of Agriculture to explain the Food Guide Pyramid and how to use it in detail (one that I highly recommend is *The Food Guide Pyramid* [USDA Home and Garden Bulletin #252]).

Meanwhile, here are two tips for using the Food Guide Pyramid effectively:

1. Keep a record of everything you eat for three days. Then compare the variety of foods and number of servings you consume with the recommendations of the Food Guide Pyramid.
2. Use the guidelines of the Food Guide Pyramid to plan menus for several days. How do these plans differ from your usual practices?

RIPPE'S RULES OF
HEALTHY EATING

As sound as the AHA/ADA Dietary Guidelines and the Food Guide Pyramid are, over the years I've still found that patients want an even simpler system that they can easily follow. So I've come up with three core concepts in nutrition that, if followed, would make us all immeasurably healthy. I call these principles Rippe's Rules of Healthy Eating.

Now I'm not saying that this system is as complete as the dietary guidelines, but it's highly practical, and many patients have told me that it's motivational and gets them started on the right track toward healthy nutrition. So if the principles we've just discussed seem too much to tackle at once, follow these three. Here goes:

Rippe's Rule 1: Eat a healthy breakfast

Breakfast is clearly the most underrated meal of the day. The cereal Wheaties is advertised as "The breakfast of Champions"! Well, if there were a champion of meals, it would be breakfast.

There are three key aspects of breakfast:

1. Eat breakfast consistently.
2. Consume an adequate number of calories.
3. Make it a low-fat meal.

Consistent healthy breakfast consumption is one of the most important rules of sound nutrition, yet it's one of the most widely violated. In our Advil Fit over Forty Standards survey of the eating habits of people over forty, 24 percent responded that they *never* eat breakfast (more than a sweet roll and coffee), 26 percent said they *seldom* eat breakfast, and only 50 percent consistently consume what I believe to be the most important meal of the day.

Why is eating breakfast so important? Because it allows you to match your calorie intake with the time that your body actually needs the calories. Once you're up and about, burning calories, your body begins to call for fuel. People who skip breakfast inevitably load up midmorning on a high-fat doughnut and a cup of coffee saturated with sugar and cream (or a similar snack). Not only are these doughnut munchers eating an enormous amount of empty calories, but they're setting themselves up for a miserable low-energy morning when their body pours out insulin to combat the sugar onslaught. When the insulin overshoots the sugar, what results is called reactive hypoglycemia, or low blood sugar. Is there any wonder why studies have shown a high correlation between obesity and breakfast skipping? This linkage is so strong that the first question I ask obese patients is what they normally eat for breakfast. A breakfast with a balance of nutrients and adequate calories keeps your body running properly.

There's an old saying among nutritionists that sums up what I think is perhaps the single most important concept in healthy nutrition: Breakfast like a king, lunch like a prince, and dinner like a pauper. Unfortunately most of us do exactly the opposite. We skip breakfast, start gathering steam around lunch, and really get down to serious eating at supper on into the evening—just in time to go to sleep and let our body store all those extra calories as fat!

A final note about breakfast: A healthy breakfast with adequate calories should also be a low-fat breakfast. Here's why.

A few years ago one of my laboratory staff conducted a study of breakfast and nutrition in college students. One group of students was given a traditional Western breakfast consisting of eggs, bacon, toast, juice, and coffee. This is a fairly typical breakfast consumed in the United States and contains about 40 percent of calories from fat. The other group was given a low-fat breakfast consisting of cereal with low-fat or skim milk, a piece of fruit, toast, juice, and coffee. At the end of three months the results were startling. The students who ate the higher-fat breakfast had slightly raised their cholesterol while the students eating the low-fat breakfast had significantly lowered theirs. Even more important, the students on the low-fat breakfast continued to eat a basically low-fat diet for the rest of the day, despite the fact that they were unsupervised. In contrast, the students on the higher-fat breakfast consumed a high-fat diet for the remainder of the day.

Why does a low-fat breakfast predict low-fat eating for the rest of the day? We don't know for sure, but I think we somehow develop a taste for fat at the beginning of the day and then continue to crave it. There's probably also an element of feeling that if we start the day with poor nutrition, why not just continue down that path?

So what's the bottom line? Eat a healthy breakfast every day. My recommendation: cereal with low-fat or skim milk; toast, bagel, or English muffin with jam; a piece of fruit; juice; and coffee, or the equivalent.

Rippe's Rule 2: Eat five servings of fruits and vegetables every day

If eating a healthy breakfast every day is the single most important nutrition health maximum, eating five servings of fruits and vegetables every day runs a close second. If we all ate five servings of fruits and vegetables on a daily basis, the incidence of heart disease, cancer, and obesity in the United States would plummet; it's one of the best things we can do to lower our risk of chronic diseases. So important is this basic concept that after years of struggling to find the right anticancer nutritional message to convey to the American public, the National Cancer Institute launched its Five Alive program to emphasize the importance of eating five servings of fruits and vegetables daily.

Why are fruits and vegetables so important in the diet? For many reasons. Fruits and vegetables are a major source of healthy, complex carbohydrates. In addition, they are loaded with antioxidants, the substances thought to play a role in decreasing heart disease and cancer by soaking up dangerous oxygen-free radicals in the body (more about these in a moment). In addition, fruits and vegetables, along with grains, are the major sources of fiber in the diet, and high-fiber consumption is clearly linked to reduced risk of colon cancer. Fruits and vegetables are loaded with vitamins, minerals, and a variety of natural substances thought to play roles in inhibiting cancer cells. The list of the healthful benefits of eating fruits and vegetables could go on and on.

Yet most of us won't let nature play this protective and healing role because we don't eat enough fruits and vegetables. The recently completed National Health and Nutrition Evaluation Survey (NHANES II) documented that 41 percent of Americans do not eat *a single serving* of fruits and vegetables on an average day. Less than 10 percent of us meet the National Cancer Institute guidelines for five servings on a daily basis.

It's a shame. Not only are we missing out on one of the great, simple, proven ways of dramatically improving our health, but we are also missing the wonderful tastes and connection with nature and the earth that prove so life-sustaining.

It doesn't have to be that way. With minimal effort we all can meet Rippe's Rule 2 and improve our health and energy by eating five servings of fruits and vegetables each day. Here's an example: Drink a tall glass of natural fruit juice and eat a banana or other piece of fruit as part of your breakfast; have a piece of fruit for lunch with your sandwich; have a salad and vegetable with dinner. You've just eaten five servings. Even better, take an extra piece of fruit for a midmorning or late-afternoon pick-me-up at work. Simple.

Rippe's Rule 3: Drink pure water

Probably the single most ignored aspect of good nutrition is proper hydration. We need to drink more water!

The human body *is* essentially water. Males are approximately 60 percent water by weight, and females approximately 55 percent. Each day each of us loses two to three quarts of water through a variety of sources; if we're physically active, add an additional quart to that total loss. So we lose up to a gallon of water on a daily basis. Now, we are absolutely obligated to consume as much as we lose. We have no choice. Remember what happens during a natural disaster, such as a hurricane or an earthquake. The most immediate and pressing nutritional need is for water, not food. Victims who are trapped die of dehydration, *not* starvation. In fact, the average individual would die in seventy-two hours if deprived of water but could live up to thirty days without food.

So how do we get the huge amount of water we need on a daily basis? From a variety of sources. Of course, we drink some as water itself. Moreover, most of the fluids we consume, such as soft drinks, coffee, tea, and juices, are more than 90 percent water. Finally, our solid food contains about 25 percent of our daily water requirement, a fact to keep in mind if you're dieting, since you need to drink extra water to prevent dehydration when food consumption declines.

So what's the problem with hydration? There are two problems really: what we drink and how much of it we drink. We're drinking the wrong fluids and not enough of the right ones. The average American adult drinks more soda pop than water. We drink an average of over five hundred cans of regular (not diet) soft drinks every year.

Since the average can of soda contains eight to twelve teaspoons of sugar, we also consume, on average, twenty-five pounds of refined sugar each year from soft drinks alone. So we could have an enormous, immediate impact on both obesity and tooth decay in our society if we substituted water for soda pop. Remember my personal saga recounted at the beginning of this chapter. The decision to switch from soda pop to water with my lunches took about a day to accomplish. The only thing I noticed was not withdrawal but actually improved energy since my body stopped having to adjust to the sugar flood.

We also don't drink *enough* water. Most of us walk around mildly dehydrated all day. Research studies from my laboratory and others have shown that water deficits of as little as a quart of water can yield substantial decreases in both physical and mental performance, and it's surprisingly easy to fall a quart behind on water consumption. In fact, if you perform moderate exercise in a temperate climate for forty-five minutes and don't drink water, you'll fall a quart behind. Even deficits smaller than a quart can also make you feel not quite at your best.

Surprisingly, our thirst is not an adequate gauge of our hydration status since it usually takes awhile to catch up and often leaves us eight to sixteen ounces behind. To combat this, I keep a bottle of water on my desk at work and sip from it periodically throughout the day. I also *always* carry water with me whenever I exercise. When I play tennis, I bring a 1.5-quart bottle of water with me onto the court. I religiously stop and drink water every five to ten minutes between games.

A few years ago I was rallying with a tennis professional at a country club near our home in the Berkshires. Between games we got into a discussion about water consumption. He had been complaining of fatigue well before the end of the long, hot days he spent on the court teaching lessons. I made a simple recommendation: He was to carry water onto the court, and drink a quart during every hour that he was out there. The next week, when I saw him, he was grinning ear to ear. "Problem solved," he exulted, "perhaps the simplest solution I've ever seen."

So what's your bottom line? Drink at least eight to sixteen ounces more pure water each day than your thirst indicates. Carry water with you when you exercise and drink liberally before, during, and after workouts. What could be easier?

BE INFORMED: READ LABELS TO HELP ACHIEVE GOOD NUTRITION GOALS

In 1993 Congress passed a law mandating new, easy-to-read labels for most of the foods we eat. I strongly support this initiative. It's hard to be certain of the composition of your diet unless you read labels.

Although there's a great deal of important information on the new labels, I think the key pieces of information are: calories, calories from fat, and amount of saturated fat contained in a serving of a particular food. For example, our first principle is to lower our consumption of saturated fat. Labels make it easy not only to see how much fat and saturated fat is in a product but also to compare similar products to determine which is lower. Ditto with calories. I always advise patients to read carefully and compare labels, and it's made an enormous difference for many of them. (Excellent pamphlets explaining the new labels are available from the American Dietetic Association, 1-800-366-1655.)

CONTROVERSIAL AND SPECIAL ISSUES IN NUTRITION

Throughout this chapter I've tried to give you an overview of the issues that I regard as holding paramount importance in the area of healthy nutrition. In a sense I've tried to give you an overview of the "forest" of nutrition. However, there are a few areas where controversies have generated intense media interest. So let's slip into the forest for a few moments to examine a few of the "trees."

Butter versus margarine

For years, we advised people to limit their intake of butter—and with good reason. Butter is loaded with saturated fat. Then, in 1994, Dr. Walter Willett, the chairman of the Department of Nutrition at the Harvard School of Public Health, wrote an article stating that the *trans*-fatty acids found in margarine were worse for your cholesterol than the saturated fats of butter.

The screams of outrage from consumers were predictable. Without getting into the particulars of Dr. Willett's argument, let me just say that he makes a compelling case to limit margarine intake. My take on the whole controversy is to limit intake of *both* margarine and butter. As I've already indicated, the monounsaturated fats, such as olive oil, are a much healthier alternative—but be careful about the calories!

Antioxidants

In 1993 two major studies linked consumption of large doses of antioxidant vitamins (vitamins C and E and beta-carotene) with substantial reductions in heart disease for both men and women. While these studies were very promising, subsequent research has not been as favorable. Two studies published in 1994 failed to show reductions in risk of cancer in individuals taking antioxidant supplements. Another study published in early 1996 failed to show that antioxidant supplements lower the risk of heart disease.

I don't believe the story on antioxidants is complete yet. Some investigators have advocated widespread use of these supplements particularly for physically active individuals. My view is that such a recommendation is premature. When patients ask me about whether or not to take antioxidants, I discuss their particular circumstances. I cannot fault individuals, especially those with personal or family histories of heart disease, for taking these supplements. However, I myself do not take them, and I do not routinely prescribe them. Several major research projects that are in progress should resolve remaining issues. My advice: Stay tuned for further developments.

Other vitamins

The field of vitamin research is one of the hottest and most productive in modern nutrition. But vitamins are also the subject of some of the most inflated and silly nutritional claims made by various health schemes and promoters. In one recent study over 50 percent of individuals who advertised themselves as nutrition counselors had no formal training in the discipline. My advice to you: Always ask to see credentials. One tip is to ask if the individual is a member of the American Dietetic Association, the major professional organization in the field.

As of this moment I cannot recommend vitamin supplements to people who are healthy and eating adequate diets. There is one exception to this. Women of childbearing potential should take a daily supplement of 400 mcg (micrograms) of folate, as should all individuals over the age of sixty-five. In this latter group folate has been shown to lower the risk of heart disease substantially.

Fish

Fish is an almost perfect food. It's a great source of high-quality protein and extremely low in fat. Yet fish consumption recently became somewhat controversial when a study showed less than expected reductions in heart disease in people who consumed large quantities. I think this is much ado about nothing. I consume fish at least three times a week and recommend it to be eaten at least twice a week by all my patients.

Coffee

Is coffee a health risk? After hundreds of studies the short answer to that question is No. Over the years concern has been raised that coffee consumption, particularly at high levels, might increase such diseases as bladder cancer and heart disease. Recent large and well-controlled studies have put these concerns to rest. The one legitimate remaining concern is the association between coffee consumption and increased risk of miscarriage. I counsel all female patients in their forties who are trying to get pregnant to eliminate coffee from their diets.

Calcium

We don't consume enough calcium. This is a common and serious problem for women of all ages but particularly after menopause, when osteoporosis becomes a major concern. The best way to slow the process of osteoporosis is to consume adequate calcium, to engage in weight bearing exercise (yet another reason to walk!), and, in some cases, for postmenopausal women, to take supplementary estrogen.

Consumption of calcium is easy to incorporate in the diet, yet over 80 percent of women over the age of forty do not consume adequate amounts. Why is this? I think it's because women don't realize that low-fat dairy products contain all the calcium of higher-fat dairy alternatives without most of the calories. In addition to dairy products, other foods high in calcium include beans, certain vegetables (such as green leafy vegetables, cauliflower, and broccoli), grains, and some fruits.

Nutrition for physically active people

I'm often asked if recreational athletes and other physically active people need special diets. The brief answer to that is no. The principles of sound nutrition apply equally to recreational athletes at all levels.

For reasons that I've never fully grasped, recreational athletes often fall prey to bizarre nutritional practices and claims. Don't fall into this trap. A diet high in carbohydrates, low in fat with moderate amounts of protein is perfect for sports-active individuals.

FINDING PEACE WITH FOOD

A few years ago, at the conclusion of a cholesterol-lowering project in my laboratory, a woman named Cecile approached me. At the start of the study she was forty-five years old and slightly overweight in addition to having a mildly elevated cholesterol of 230 mg/dl. More important, she had terrible nutritional habits. Her diet of simple-to-prepare cheese sandwiches for lunch and frequent red meat for dinner meant that over 50 percent of her calories came from fat, much of it saturated. Just lowering her fat consumption had effortlessly dropped her weight and cholesterol level and elevated her energy.

As she approached me, she had a tear in her eye. I'll never forget what she said. "Thank you," she exclaimed, "not just for helping me lose weight and lower my cholesterol but for finally helping me find peace with food."

Food is joy, nutrition, celebration, taste, sharing—the sustenance of life. My fondest wish for all of us is that we join Cecile in finding "peace with food."

CHAPTER 13

HEALTHY WEIGHT MANAGEMENT

SHARON

Sharon plunked down on the seat beside me. "I'm tired," she said. "Physically tired, emotionally tired, tired of being overweight, and just plain tired of being tired."

Sharon had come to my laboratory in response to a notice we had published in a local newspaper announcing the start of a research study exploring healthy weight loss. This was the third major project we had conducted in this vast and vital area, so the response shouldn't have surprised me, but it always did.

We were looking for eighty individuals who were between 20 and 40 percent above desirable weight who would be willing to participate in a research trial exploring the weight loss and body composition changes along with physical and psychological consequences of a twelve-week program of low-fat eating, exercise, and group support. As soon as the papers hit the streets, the phone began to ring—over four hundred calls in the first eight hours. When people couldn't get through to the lab via telephone, they walked in through the front door clutching the notice. It was impossible to conduct other lab business for the next two days.

"I've tried every diet in the book." Sharon continued. "I've been on the grapefruit diet, the Atkins diet, the low-fat diet, the high-protein diet—you name it, I've been on it!" She paused. "I'm too fat. I don't like this weight, and I know it's not healthy. But mostly I don't like how I feel, and I'm tired of failing."

Even though Sharon had never participated in one of our studies and had never seen me as a patient, I knew her very well. She was one of the best nurses in our coronary care unit, where we had collaborated caring for desperately ill patients for the better part of a decade. Sharon was fifty-six years old. She had been overweight for the entire time I knew her. As she told me her story, it was clear that she hadn't always been overweight but, like so many others, had slowly drifted into a pattern where weight gain was almost inevitable.

During nursing school Sharon weighed between 120 and 125 pounds—an excellent weight for her five-foot-five-inch height. She had married immediately after graduation and adopted a lifestyle that began to contribute to a slow accretion of pounds. She worked a stressful job, had the responsibilities of a new home, entertained, and with her husband, Tony, ate out three or four times a week. Mostly she didn't pay attention, and by her mid-twenties she weighed 130 pounds, size six was history. She was now a solid size eight, but so were all her friends, and her husband, who had also gained weight, loved the way she looked.

The dramatic change came with the birth of Sarah, her first child. Sharon gained 30 pounds during the pregnancy—a perfectly reasonable amount—but afterward shed only 18 pounds. She now tipped the scales at 142. Two more children brought similar results, and when she was forty-two, the scales read 164 pounds. She looked and felt positively matronly.

This was also the beginning of Sharon's food torture. Throughout her forties she tried diet after diet, throwing herself into food prison for periods of up to six months, only to break out on a food rampage of several weeks that put back every pound she had struggled so mightily to remove. Finally, at the age of fifty, she gave up. "I decided I was fat, but what the hell. I didn't like it, but I wasn't willing to put up with the constant misery and repeated failures of trying to lose the weight. I decided that this was who I was and so be it. I had three lovely children and two grandchildren. I was a grandmother, so it was okay to look like one!"

So why the change of heart? Why was she sitting next to me volunteering for a weight loss study—and one that required exercise? Because she was smart, because she kept on listening and reading and became convinced that she was destroying her health, and because she was tired of being fat and tired of being tired.

I explained to Sharon, as I had already to twenty previous volunteers that morning, that she had only a 50 percent chance of being assigned to the "intervention" group, which would receive the diet, exercise, and group support program. The other 50 percent would constitute a "control" group to assure the scientific validity of the research trial. Unlike many of the previous volunteers, Sharon was versed in the need to avoid bias through the random selection process and readily agreed to participate in the process. "I feel lucky," she said. And she was; she *did* get randomly assigned to the intervention group. (In fairness, I should tell you that we always offer subjects in the control group the opportunity to participate in the intervention program once the original research project is completed.)

Sharon's original data offered no real surprises. She was too fat, poorly conditioned, and anxious—*just like one third of all adults in the United States*. Her body fat was 34 percent, her Body Mass Index (BMI) was 27.5, her aerobic capacity was a below-average 28 ml/kg/min, and her daily calorie consumption was slightly elevated at 2,570 kcal/day with a whopping 42 percent of calories from fat. Sharon also underwent extensive psychological testing since as part of the study since treating the body without enlisting the mind is a recipe for failure in any weight loss program. We found that she was anxious and mildly depressed, lacked confidence in her physical ability, and had below-average measurements of physical and mental components of quality of life. No surprises here. Sharon tested just the way she looked, someone who was overweight, underconditioned, and unhappy with her life.

What happened to Sharon over the next month was nothing short of miraculous. She caught fire. In fact, she got into the program in such a big way that we had to slow her down. During the first two weeks she lost four pounds each week—much more than the one to two pounds a week we consider safe, reasonable, and sustainable. We sat her down, convinced her to add more calories back to her diet, and reminded her that weight management is a race won by the tortoise, not the hare. The goal is to achieve long-term control of the lifestyle factors that can make or break anyone's attempt to control weight.

At the end of twelve weeks Sharon was a new woman. She had lost eighteen pounds. Significantly, 100 percent of the weight she lost was fat; her exercise program had enabled her to maintain her all-important lean muscle tissue. Her body fat had dipped to 25 percent, and her aerobic capacity had shot up 20 percent to 33 ml/kg/min—a result of her fitness walking program of three miles a day, six days a week. ("Never on Sunday!" she had joked with me.) Her fat intake was down to 28 percent of total calories, which had declined to eighteen hundred a day—built back slowly from the twelve hundred a day she had maintained the first ten weeks of the study. Most important, Sharon's mood and approach to her body and the world had changed dramatically. "My energy and confidence are higher than they've ever been in my life," she exulted, and the results on our battery of psychological tests confirmed her assessment.

Six months later, when I saw Sharon in my office for a follow-up, she had lost another ten pounds and found a new life. It was no longer surprising to her that she walked almost every day; it was now part of her life—a part she couldn't imagine living without.

THE BAD NEWS AND GOOD NEWS OF OBESITY

Obesity in the United States is the classic good news, bad news situation. The predicament Sharon found herself in—slow persistent weight gain throughout the middle years—happens all too commonly in our country. In fact, obesity has exploded into an epidemic of immense proportions. Each year over three hundred thousand preventable deaths occur because Americans are overweight, and the number is rapidly growing. Obesity is currently the second leading cause of preventable death in the United States behind cigarette smoking. However, at the current rate of growth it will surpass smoking as the number one cause of preventable death in the United States by the year 2000.

I'd like to report that we've recognized this public health menace and are moving rapidly to correct the problem. Unfortunately just the opposite is true! Even though the negative health consequences of obesity have now become clear to the medical community, the public doesn't seem to understand the links between weight and health. In its most recent findings the National Health and Nutrition Evaluation Survey (NHANES) reported that in the period between 1980 and 1990 the incidence of obesity in the United States *grew* by a shocking 31 percent. For both sexes and in all racial groups, one out of every three adults in the United States is now clinically obese—fat to a level that his or her health is placed in serious jeopardy. That's the bad news side of the equation.

On the good news side, we have wonderful information that even small amounts of weight loss, if sustained over time, can yield significant health benefits, and the techniques for achieving these results are well within each of our grasps. Yet if you've had the problem of weight gain in your life, you know it can be frustratingly difficult to reverse. In this chapter I'm going to show you how to end this issue in your life— simply, healthfully, and for good.

THE WEIGHT AND HEALTH CONNECTION

Why do I care so much about the weight and health connection? Because the linkage is so strong, it's so easy to take the simple steps to control your weight and improve your health, yet few people truly understand how their increased weight is harming their health. Increased weight has been clearly associated with increased risk of heart disease, certain forms of cancer, diabetes, osteoarthritis, and many other conditions. Let's look at a few of these.

Cardiovascular disease

Increased weight has been associated with coronary artery disease in both men and women. This negative relationship occurs through two mechanisms. First, increased weight elevates blood pressure and cholesterol levels, both of which are established risk factors for coronary heart disease. Second, increased weight carries an independent connection with increased heart disease beyond elevating risk factors.

The first thing I tell an overweight individual with coronary artery disease, high blood pressure, or elevated cholesterol is that she or he must lose weight. Often it's all a person needs to bring all these problems under control. Data from the Framingham Heart Study and the

Nurses' Health Study, both enormous and well-conducted studies, show that even weight gains as small as fifteen to twenty pounds during adulthood substantially increase the risk of heart disease. Unfortunately this relationship follows the classic dose-response curve—that is, the higher your weight, the higher your risk. At the weight that Sharon had reached, her risk of heart disease was more than doubled.

Cancer

The relationship between being overweight and increased risk of cancer is not as obvious as the risk of heart disease, but it's just as real. In the Nurse's Health Study, the research into more than one hundred thousand female nurses who have now been followed for more than twenty years, most of the increased risk of death is associated with increased risk of cancer. In fact, 80 percent of all the deaths in this study of middle-aged women came from cancer, and there was a direct linkage to overweight. Once again, the more overweight the individual, the greater the risk of cancer—particularly of the colon or breast. By the time a woman has a BMI of over 30 (in Sharon's case this would mean a weight of 180 pounds at her five feet five inches) her risk of cancer quadruples. And there is no reason to doubt that the same general relationship exists for males.

No one knows for sure how cancer and obesity are linked, but most theories are based on hormonal changes that occur as the result of the increased presence and size of fat cells.

Diabetes

Adult-onset diabetes mellitus, the type of diabetes that 95 percent of diabetics have, is strongly linked to obesity. In fact, one of the best preventive measures you can take to minimize your risk of diabetes is to maintain a normal body weight, and one of the most important steps in the treatment of adult-onset diabetes is to lose weight.

The linkage between adult-onset diabetes and obesity seems to be through insulin resistance. Individuals who have this condition are resistant to their bodies' own insulin, and obesity makes them even more so.

Osteoarthritis

Overweight individuals are much more prone to osteoarthritis, the most common form of arthritis, than people who maintain desirable weight. This linkage comes largely through the increased pounding on the bones and joints from the extra pounds, but there is probably a biochemical link through the fat cells as well.

This list of associated disease states could go on and on, but here's my point. Being overweight should be viewed not as a *vanity* issue but as a *health* issue. And the simple steps I'm going to propose to counteract this problem are some of the smartest health steps you'll ever take.

HOW MUCH WEIGHT IS TOO MUCH WEIGHT?

Perhaps a few definitions are in order. When I say "obese," I am talking about carrying at least 20 percent more weight (typically fat weight) than is desirable for your height. This clinical definition describes a much lower weight gain than most people associate with the term "obese," which most of us tend to think describes someone other than us. We need to realize, however, that only "a few" pounds too much—as little as fifteen to thirty—can make a big difference. In medical practices, we typically determine obesity by using the Body Mass Index (BMI), as you did when you took the Fit over Forty Tests. Individuals who have BMIs greater than 27 are defined as being clinically obese, although as we've begun to learn, even levels of weight below a BMI of 27 can begin to accelerate the risks of various medical problems. So what weight's right for you?

HEALTHY WEIGHT, HEALTHIER WEIGHT, AND OPTIMAL WEIGHT

There has been a great deal of controversy about what constitutes a healthy weight, and while we in the medical community have tried to understand the data and debate our differences, I'm afraid we've confused a lot of people. Let me give you an example.

In 1993 the USDA published new tables that told people it was all right to be a little heavier than previous tables had indicated. These new tables really featured two new concepts. First, they allowed people to be about twenty pounds heavier than previous tables at any given height and still fall within the healthy weight range. Second, they established an age cutoff of thirty-five years old. Over the age of thirty-five the healthy weight range was liberalized even further to allow us older individuals to be even a little heavier and stay within this range. So far, so good. The government was acting with the best information at its disposal to try to help us all understand the links between weight and health. Unfortunately the publication of these new tables really represented the "calm before the storm." In 1994 and 1995 my friends Dr. Ralph Paffenbarger and Dr. JoAnn Manson published a series of excellent papers showing that the government tables were far too liberal. Their studies, based on huge population samples of men and women, showed that leaner was better down to very low levels of weight when it came to lowering the risk of developing chronic disease. By now everyone was thoroughly confused.

I'll never forget Sharon striding up to me in the hall after the study by Dr. Manson was published. Sharon had a vested interest in this study not only because of her own successful weight loss efforts but also because the study had been conducted in a group of over one hundred thousand female nurses.

"I'd call this the Barbie study," she protested, waving the weight and height tables from the study reprinted that day in *The Boston Globe*. I had to admit she had a point. According to the study, the lowest risk of dying occurred in those nurses who had a very slender Body Mass Index of less than 19. To put that in perspective, for a woman of Sharon's height of five feet five inches, the lowest mortality was found in people who weighed less than 119 pounds. This comprises less than 10 percent of women of this height in the United States or, as Sharon put it, "the Barbies of the world."

So what are we to make of this whole debate and controversy? I think the appropriate response is fairly straightforward and can be explained by three related concepts: *healthy weight, healthier weight,* and *optimum weight*. Each of us has a weight range that is basically healthy for us. I call this our healthy weight. This weight varies according to our height and somewhat to our frame size (although be careful about the concept of frame size since I've never met an overweight person who didn't argue that he or she had a "large" frame). The old weight tables were too restrictive in terms of healthy weight, while the USDA tables of 1993 were too liberal. My best advice: Keep your BMI below 25 to maintain healthy weight (BMI tables are in Chapter 3).

In addition to the healthy weight that each of us has, we each have a healthier weight, regardless of what our current weight is. The good news here is that there is now excellent evidence that even if your weight has drifted up forty to sixty pounds over the years, if you lose ten to fifteen pounds and keep it off, your risk of chronic disease declines precipitously.

Finally, there is an optimum weight for each of us. This constitutes the weight at which our risks for chronic disease are driven to an absolute minimum. For most of us, that optimum weight may be far below what we realistically can or even want to achieve. But the good news is that higher weights can be healthy or at least healthier.

Let's look at these concepts through Sharon's eyes. When she joined our research study, she weighed 164 pounds. At her five feet five inches that gave her an unhealthy BMI of 27.5. By our definition she was obese. She lost 18 pounds in the study, another 10 in the next six months, and 4 more, which she had managed to keep off for the next three years. Today, at 132 pounds, her BMI is a healthy 22, and this weight is healthier than her original 164. Now her optimal weight may be a BMI of less than 19 or a weight of 119, but neither she nor I have this as a goal for her. She doesn't have to look like Barbie to be healthy and healthier than she was before.

EFFECTIVE WEIGHT MANAGEMENT

The principles of effective weight management have become increasingly clear over the last decade as many research laboratories, including mine, have given major emphasis to the issue. What we've learned establishes some core principles in this area that lead to practical daily plans. Let's look at them.

Principle 1: You must burn more calories than you take in

This, of course, is somewhat obvious, but it's absolutely the fundamental truth in weight loss and weight management. If you have gained weight in the middle years, it's because you've consistently taken in more calories than you've consumed.

How does this happen? Most people who experience middle-age spread get it because over the years, without noticing, they've slowly stopped exercising, stopped taking walks, and, in general, started leading more sedentary lives. As a result, the energy equation—the relationship between calories taken in and calories expended—has slowly tipped out of their favor, and it doesn't take much of an imbalance to create an enormous problem. If you consume one more cookie each day than you burn through your daily activities, at the end of one year you will have gained ten pounds.

To lose weight effectively, you must tip the energy equation in your favor. There are only three ways to do this: dieting (decreasing the number of calories you consume each day), exercise (increasing the number of calories you burn), and a combination of diet and exercise.

Numerous studies have come to one inescapable conclusion: The *only* effective solution for healthy weight loss and permanent weight management is the combination of diet and exercise. The Fit over Forty Eating Plan for Weight Management, which I'll share with you in a few pages, has been designed to complement your Fit over Forty Walking (or other) Program to help you achieve such permanent weight management.

Principle 2: It is impossible to achieve permanent weight management without consistent exercise

I've already told you that attention to both diet and regular exercise are important, but over the years I've come to believe that regular exercise is paramount. Recently researchers at Rockefeller University showed that individuals who tried to gain or lose weight were resisted every step of the way by their bodies. In other words, when people purposefully tried to gain weight, their metabolism sped up to resist this change. When people tried to lose weight, their metabolism slowed down to resist this change.

This study provided further evidence of what is called the set point theory, according to which, the body will rigorously defend a certain set point of weight—usually the highest stable weight.

What does the set point theory have to do with exercise? Everything! When you try to lose weight, your metabolism slows down to resist you, and the *only* healthy and effective way to counteract this is to increase the calories you burn through exercise. Unless you are willing to increase the amount of physical activity in your life, you will *never* achieve lifelong weight management. I've seen this statement to be true for hundreds of people. After all, you can't fight Mother Nature.

Principle 3: Adopt a lifelong strategy
for what is a lifelong problem

The most common problem that people experience in weight management, and the major reason for failure, are that they try short-term fixes for what is for almost everyone a lifelong problem. Success in weight management requires an honest appraisal of your circumstances. For me it was abandoning my high-fat, high-calorie lunches. For Sharon it was attention to diet combined with daily walking. Effective weight management requires a lifelong commitment to changing the lifestyle habits that caused the problem in the first place. Short-term approaches don't work.

So what's the answer? Living fully, consciously, and in the present. Paying attention to the composition of your diet and, most important, your daily exercise is the only effective way to achieve permanent weight management. It *is* simple. Yes, I know, the devil is in the details, but I've seen too many people succeed with these simple measures to doubt their power.

MASTERING THE MIND-SET

Weight gain is the classic mind-body problem. Unfortunately many individuals, including many in the medical profession, have made the fundamental error of treating only the body. When we overeat and underexercise, we are waging war on our bodies. Why would anyone consciously do this? I think it comes more from spiritual hunger than from the physical need for calories. After all, eating is one of the most highly effective ways to quell anxiety. Why do you think people snack before going to bed?

My point here is that if you've had a problem with weight gain or have failed with previous attempts to lose and permanently keep off extra weight, I'll guarantee you it's because the problem was framed as a physical one rather than as a mind-body issue. This approach compounds the problem. People who follow short-term diets throw themselves in food prison. Not only are they hungry and preoccupied with food all the time, but they're also depressed. They're fighting both mind and body.

There is a good news side to this situation. Once you commit to the simple, fundamental lifestyle changes of eating mindfully and engaging in enjoyable physical activity, the mind-body aspects of weight management start working for you rather than against you. The response that Sharon had, increased energy and confidence and a renewed joy for life, is the universal response I've seen in individuals who commit to these fundamental changes. Once you've experienced that, both your mind and body are finally satisfied, and you'll never go back.

WHAT ABOUT THE OBESITY GENE?

In December 1994 researchers in New York announced the discovery of a gene that caused obesity in a particular strain of mice. Their work was quickly followed by demonstration that the hormone (leptin) regulated by this gene caused dramatic weight loss in these mice. Another group of researchers in Massachusetts quickly reported a second obesity gene in another type of mouse. In both instances scientists believed that similar genes are found in humans.

After the first announcement of the mouse obesity gene, Charlotte, one of my patients who has struggled with a lifelong obesity problem, called me. "Doc, I've finally figured it out!" she exclaimed. "It's my genes! No wonder I can't keep weight off."

Well . . . maybe. There is no question that there is a powerful genetic component to obesity. Numerous studies have now shown that some people are more predisposed to weight gain than others. And I believe that the research into mouse obesity genes carries enormous potential to help us ultimately understand and treat obesity in humans. But it's not the complete answer.

I share the belief of most other scientists in this field that genetics accounts for approximately 60 percent of the underlying cause of obesity. That still leaves an incredible 40 percent for the daily lifestyle decisions we all make. Think about it for a moment. The incidence of obesity shot up 31 percent between 1980 and 1990, yet it takes thousands of years for the gene pool to shift even slightly. We didn't all of a sudden grow 31 percent more obesity genes.

One more thing about the obesity gene: Even under the most optimistic scenario, products that might help with human obesity will not be available for five to ten years, and then, *if* they work, they're only going to be part of the solution.

WHAT ABOUT DRUGS?

Every Wednesday evening, along with my colleagues Gayle Gardner and Dr. Lou Aronne, I conduct a national medical call-in show for the Television Food Network. Almost invariably someone will call wanting to discuss drug therapy for obesity.

Let me give you my view on this. A number of drugs that hold some promise to assist in weight loss have been introduced over the past five years. One combination that has been demonstrated effective in short-term trials is phentermine combined with fenfluramine (the so-called phen-fen combination). For some people this has effectively helped with loss of about 10 percent of body weight. Even newer drugs that also offer promise to assist in weight control are on the horizon. Many of these drugs act on brain chemistry and the sense of satiety, or fullness, although the mechanisms are varied.

While there may be some role for drug therapy in the treatment of obesity, I believe it will be for the minority of individuals, and as research dictates, even in these it may be effective only in conjunction with the lifestyle measures already discussed. The history of medicine is littered with drug therapies that showed some promise but failed as the sole treatment for problems that are as complicated as obesity.

THE FIT OVER FORTY EATING PLAN
FOR WEIGHT MANAGEMENT

With this informational foundation in place, you're now ready to design your personal eating plan to achieve and maintain a healthy weight. The Fit over Forty Eating Plan has two goals: (1) to help you reach your weight loss goals and (2) to help you develop new eating habits and lifestyle practices that will continue to work for you and not against you. To do that, you need a way to organize a convenient weight loss "diet" and, without carrying around a pocket computer, to follow the healthy nutritional practices discussed in the last chapter. You need a plan that's flexible and fits your tastes, schedule, and lifestyle. You also need a plan that doesn't take away the natural enjoyment of food and the fellowship that are part of mealtimes.

To provide all these benefits, the Fit over Forty Eating Plan uses a food exchange system rather than calorie counting. This system organizes all food into six exchange categories (similar to those of the Food Guide Pyramid): starches/bread, meats/protein, vegetables, fruits, milk, fat. Within each category a single food exchange contains approximately the same amount of calories and grams of carbohydrates, protein, or fat, allowing you to substitute one food for another as you like while ensuring that you are getting the nutrients and calories you need to reach your weight loss goals. With a little practice, using food exchanges becomes a comfortable habit, something you need never think about, helping you maintain your weight at healthy levels for the rest of your life.

Although you may have to give yourself a week or two to become accustomed to thinking about your meals and your food portions a little differently, I think you'll find that this approach is very effective. The Fit over Forty Eating Plan is adapted from a program I have used extensively in my laboratory and medical practice and published in *The Exercise Exchange Program*. In addition to this research, the program draws on the Food Exchange Lists and meal planning system originally designed and approved by the American Diabetes Association and American Dietetic Association for diabetics and others who had to follow special diets but long since proved, because of their practicality, flexibility, and sound nutritional base, to work very well for anyone. The system works because it doesn't tell you what you must eat but provides a way of managing food to fit your tastes and lifestyle. At the same time it supplies a framework designed to help you meet these goals of sound weight loss management: nutritional balance and variety, low-fat content, and portion control. Let me also remind you that it's designed to be used in conjunction with your Fit over Forty Personal Fitness Program—the only sure route to long-term weight management.

To help you get started on the Fit over Forty Eating Plan, I've provided these guides:

- Fit over Forty Meal Plans for 1,200-, 1,500-, and 1,800-calorie diets
- A description of the food exchanges and tips on their use
- Fit over Forty Weekly Exchange Checklist

For more information you'll find detailed Food Exchange Lists and sample Seven-Day Fit over Forty Menu Plans in the Appendix.

Now with the clairvoyance of long experience, I know what you're thinking: Sure sounds complex, no matter what he says. Not really.

Give yourself a little time—commit to following through with at least a twelve-week eating plan in conjunction with your exercise plan—and I think you'll find that this is another of those useful guide maps I promised you.

One final comment: Many people find group support very helpful for weight loss. Over the years my laboratory has worked with Weight Watchers International. We have found its weight loss principles and plans highly effective; they're based on concepts very similar to the ones we've developed in our laboratory, including the food exchange system. When my patients inquire about a weight loss program that includes group support, I always refer them to Weight Watchers.

THE FIT OVER FORTY MEAL PLANS

The Fit over Forty Eating Plan is designed to help you lose one half to one pound per week—the recommended goal—using a meal plan of 1,200, 1,500, or 1,800 calories per day. Each meal plan provides a set number of exchanges in each category and some open calories for you to use any way you like (as long as you go slow on the fats). Within this set number of exchanges, you may arrange the exchanges any way you like during the day and select any foods you like within the food categories. In this way the Fit over Forty Eating Plan provides a framework on which you design your own eating plan. Let's look at the plans, and then I'll show you how to select the one that is appropriate for you.

1,200-CALORIE MEAL PLAN

Exchanges:	4 meat	3 fruit
	4 starch/bread	3 fat
	3 vegetable	2 milk
Open calories: 80		

1,500-CALORIE MEAL PLAN

Exchanges:	5 meat	4 fruit
	5 starch/bread	3 fat
	3 vegetable	2 milk
Open calories: 200		

1,800-CALORIE MEAL PLAN

Exchanges:	6 meat	4 fruit
	6 starch/bread	4 fat
	4 vegetable	2 milk
Open calories: 300		

Selecting the right plan

To calculate which plan is appropriate for you, multiply your present body weight by 10 to reach the calories you need. For example, if you now weigh 180 pounds, multiply 180 by 10 to equal 1,800 calories. If your calorie need places you in between these plans, simply add or subtract from the open calories in the nearest standard plan to reach your goal. Here are some samples for in-between numbers to show you how:

1,300 calories: Use the 1,200-calorie plan, and add another 100 open calories.

1,400 calories: Use the 1,500-calorie plan, but subtract 100 open calories.

1,600 calories: Add another 100 open calories to the 1,500-calorie plan, or if you want more guidance from the exchange structure, subtract 200 calories from the 1,800-calorie plan.

1,700 calories: Subtract 100 open calories from the 1,800-calorie plan.

1,900 calories: Add one starch/bread exchange to the 1,800-calorie plan.

More than 1,900 calories: Add one meat, one starch/bread, and one fruit exchange to the 1,800-calorie plan.

Tips for Using the Meal Plans

Use the meal plans to plan ahead. In the first few weeks, as you get used to
   the food exchange approach, take the time to plan your meals
   ahead as much as possible. You may find the sample menus starting on page 298 helpful. Planning ahead helps make the idea of
   food exchanges second nature and gives you a better chance to
   adapt the approach to your needs. For example, if you plan to eat
   out for dinner but are not sure where, saving some starch and fat
   exchanges and your open calories for the evening is probably
   smart, so for lunch you might have a mixed vegetable salad topped
   by one meat exchange of turkey or lean ham and a piece of fruit,
   rather than use up more bread and meat exchanges in a sandwich.

Watch for hidden fats: Hidden fats in prepared foods can sabotage your
   goals to keep your calories from fat under 30 percent. So read the
   labels carefully in products you purchase to eat at home, and be
   alert when you eat out. For example, if you load on the high-fat regular salad dressings at the salad bar rather than choose a modest
   serving of the reduced-calorie dressing, you can blow your fat
   exchanges for a whole week.

Give yourself time. Don't weigh yourself more than once a week, if that,
   and give your plan at least four weeks before you modify it up or
   down to adjust for weight loss that is too rapid or too slow.

*Don't forget that the Fit over Forty Eating Plan was designed to be used in
   conjunction with an exercise program.* Following only the eating plan
   without the exercise plan will lead to frustration and failure.

THE FOOD EXCHANGES AND HOW TO USE THEM

Below are each of the six food exchange categories and sample exchanges. With these basics you can start to plan and implement your daily food plan. If you need more than the basics, however, complete Food Exchange Lists that detail the specific foods and quantities in each category are on page 322, in the Appendix.

Starch/Bread Exchanges

1 exchange	=	½ cup cereal, cooked pasta or cooked grain (rice, bulgur, etc.)
		1 ounce bread or bread product
		½ cup starchy vegetables, such as corn, mashed potatoes, cooked dried peas, and beans
		3 ounces baked potato
	=	80 calories
	=	15 grams carbohydrates, 3 grams protein, trace fat

Add a fat exchange to: biscuit (2.5 inches), corn bread (2-inch-square), waffle or pancake (4 inches), or 10 french fries

Meat/Protein Exchanges

1 exchange	=	1 ounce lean meat or medium fat meat or fish
		1 ounce part-skim diet cheese
		¼ cup cottage cheese, part-skim ricotta
		¼ cup canned water-packed tuna, salmon
		1 egg
	=	55–70 calories
	=	7 grams protein, 3–5 grams fat

Add a fat exchange for each 1-ounce exchange of high-fat meats, such as prime beef, beef or pork ribs, sausage, or luncheon meat, such as salami or bologna.

Vegetable Exchanges

1 exchange　　=　　½ cup cooked vegetables or vegetable juice

　　　　　　　　　　1 cup raw vegetables

　　　　　　　=　　25 calories

　　　　　　　=　　5 grams carbohydrates, 3 grams protein

Fruit Exchanges

1 exchange　　=　　½ cup fresh fruit or fruit juice

　　　　　　　　　　¼ cup dried fruit

　　　　　　　=　　60 calories

　　　　　　　=　　15 grams carbohydrates

Tip: Canned fruit should be packed in juice, not heavy or light syrup.

Milk Exchanges

1 exchange　　=　　1 cup skim or 1 percent milk, buttermilk

　　　　　　　　　　1 cup nonfat yogurt

　　　　　　　=　　90 calories

　　　　　　　=　　12 grams carbohydrates, 8 grams protein, trace to 3 grams fat

Add a fat exchange for 1 cup 2 percent or whole milk.

Fat Exchanges

1 exchange　　=　　quantity varies greatly depending on product but samples include:

　　　　　　　　　　1 teaspoon butter/margarine

　　　　　　　　　　1 teaspoon oil

　　　　　　　　　　1 teaspoon regular mayonnaise

　　　　　　　　　　2 tablespoon light cream or sour cream

　　　　　　　　　　1 tablespoon heavy (whipping) cream

　　　　　　　　　　1 slice bacon

　　　　　　　=　　45 calories

　　　　　　　=　　5 grams of fat

Tip: High-fat foods like nuts, salad dressings, olives, and avocados fall into this category. Go sparingly.

Free Foods

You may eat these without counting them as an exchange: noncalorie drinks, such as tea, coffee, or sugar-free soda; herbs and spices; salad greens, and such vegetables as raw celery, radishes, cabbage, cucumbers, and mushrooms; 1 tablespoon ketchup, salsa, horseradish, mustard, vinegar.

Alcohol

Since the idea is to be flexible and practical, here are appropriate exchanges for those who would like a glass of wine with dinner or an occasional beer with friends. The watchword, however, is *moderation* because alcohol's calories have little nutritive value as well as because of the physiological and psychological dangers of imbibing too much. Furthermore, alcohol is *loaded* with calories, and unless you pay attention to the amount you consume, it can torpedo the best-laid diet plans.

2 fat exchanges	=	4 ounces wine, 12 ounces light beer, or 1.5 ounces (1 shot) liquor
1 starch, 2 fat exchanges	=	12 ounces regular beer

Combination Foods

Combination foods, such as casseroles or mixed stir-fries or pasta dishes, are a regular feature of most menus and part of the fun of eating. Usually you can estimate exchanges, particularly if you make the dish from scratch or consult the label on the box, but sometimes the mix is so mysterious you haven't any idea. The Food Exchange Lists on page 322 can give you a clue. Remember to be alert for combination dishes that are prepared with a lot of oil or fats or include such high-fat ingredients as cream sauces, cheese, and high-fat meats.

Tips on using the exchanges: Making exchanges within six categories may seem a lot to learn at first, but if you'll study them a moment, you will see that most portion sizes within a category are very similar. With a little planning and practice you'll soon remember just what they are. It may also help to visualize the exchange sizes. For example, if you can't picture the size of a half cup (a common exchange measure), get the half cup measure out of the kitchen drawer and study it, or actually measure your portions at one meal at home and study the size. As you go along, you'll develop your own rules of thumb that work for you. For example, three ounces of cooked meat (three meat exchanges) is about the size of a cooked "quarter pounder" beef patty or the palm of your hand.

FIT OVER FORTY EATING PLAN WEEKLY EXCHANGE CHECKLIST

The easiest way to keep track of your eating plan is to check off the day's exchanges as you consume them. Make photocopies of this handy form, and keep one in your wallet, pocket, or daily planner—whatever's most convenient for you.

FIT OVER FORTY WEEKLY EXCHANGE CHECKLIST
1,200-CALORIE MEAL PLAN

No. Exchanges	Exchange	Mon	Tues	Wed	Thurs	Fri	Sat	Sun
4	Starch							
4	Meat							
3	Veg.							
3	Fruit							
2	Milk							
3	Fat							
80	Open cal.							

FIT OVER FORTY WEEKLY EXCHANGE CHECKLIST
1,500-CALORIE MEAL PLAN

No. Exchanges	Exchange	Mon	Tues	Wed	Thurs	Fri	Sat	Sun
5	Starch							
5	Meat							
3	Veg.							
4	Fruit							
2	Milk							
3	Fat							
200	Open cal.							

FIT OVER FORTY WEEKLY EXCHANGE CHECKLIST
1,800-CALORIE MEAL PLAN

No. Exchanges	Exchange	Mon	Tues	Wed	Thurs	Fri	Sat	Sun
6	Starch							
6	Meat							
4	Veg.							
4	Fruit							
2	Milk							
4	Fat							
300	Open cal.							

PEACE IN OUR TIME

A few years ago at a conference a colleague asked for my assessment of future directions in the research for exercise and nutrition. "That's easy," I responded. "There will continue to be vigorous research in both areas, but I see them coming closer and closer together under the umbrella of positive lifestyle. And the playing field where research in nutrition and exercise come together will be called weight management."

Today, a few years later, I stand by this statement. The only thing I didn't predict was the rapid and dangerous rise in the incidence of obesity in our country. You know by now that I believe health is about daily decisions and habits—those things we do each day that determine whether we are at peace or not with ourselves. I've told you that exercise is the way to find peace with our bodies. And proper nutrition is the process of coming to peace with food.

Let's not make weight management too difficult. If we take the simple steps to find peace with our bodies and peace with food, the war that most people wage with weight all their lives is over and we'll each find peace in our time.

PART FOUR

FIT OVER FORTY NO MATTER WHAT

CHAPTER 14

FITNESS AND AGING: TIPS FOR STAYING IN THE GAME FOR THE REST OF YOUR LIFE

SEASONS

I am sitting at my desk in our Berkshire home overlooking our fields as I have done a thousand times or more over the past decade since I purchased the house as a writing, reading, walk-in-the-woods getaway. The weather has grown colder. It is mid-October, a time in New England when frost is in the air. The harvest is long since in from all the truck farms in our area, and the multihued orange and red and yellow leaves from our maples are swirling on light breezes as they gently pirouette toward the ground.

I feel good, probably better than I have ever felt in my life, and I am thinking about seasons. Fifteen months ago I married a beautiful woman eleven years my junior, and now she's carrying our first baby. We sandwich forty, she and I, and while in some ways we approach the age denoted by that number in very similar ways, in others our perspective is quite different.

I am in early August of my life, I have decided, and she is in mid-June. This past summer I turned forty-eight. As I point toward fifty, my life seems better, fuller, more understandable than ever before. Unless I really miss my guess, I am also in the second half of my life—late summer—and facing the challenges and opportunities presented by that incredibly rich season. While I may not yet be ready for harvest, I am certainly thinking about fall in my own life and determined that it will come to me as John Berryman wrote, "as a prize."'

AGING, FUNCTION, AND HEALTH

Over the past twenty years in medicine and research I have had the privilege of caring for and conducting research projects involving several thousand individuals over the age of forty. While their histories, backgrounds, hopes, fears, and aspirations are as different as the people themselves, several themes have become abundantly clear.

First, after we pass forty, the issue of aging becomes a factor in almost everything we do. Whether we are forty-five, fifty-five, or sixty-five, by this point in our lives we recognize that we will not live forever, and everyone, in one way or another, factors that realization into his or her life. Second, after forty, health and function become dominant concerns. In my experience, people over forty do not want to turn back the clock or even stop aging; what most people want is to maintain good health, feel good about and happy with their lives, and function at their absolute peak—for whatever age they are. And the good news is that you can, just like my friend Mary.

MARY

I first heard about Mary from a staff researcher working on our first project to establish age- and sex-specific standards for the One-Mile Walk Test. At sixty-eight Mary just squeaked in under the cutoff line of age sixty-nine, but her walking performance was anything but marginal. She blasted through the mile in twelve minutes and thirty-four seconds, setting an age and sex walking record for women in their sixties that still stands in my laboratory. In fact, her time put her in the "excellent" category for women in their thirties.

Two months later we met when she showed up as a patient in my office. Her goal was simple, she stated: She was unwilling to go quietly into the night.

"After teaching briefly, I married and had my children early," Mary said, "so by the age of fifty-five my husband and I were looking at an empty nest. For a few years I played golf, gardened, and dabbled in tennis and took vacations with my husband. It all sounded good, but it was driving me nuts. I felt bored and too old for my age. I decided I had to take a stand. For the past ten years I've been on a one-woman campaign to prevent myself from becoming a little old lady."

As part of her campaign, Mary had joined a local health club, started volunteer work at a local community center for troubled children, and enrolled in night school to become recertified as a teacher.

Quickly her life began to change. The health club membership started paying dividends first. After an initial period of soreness she gradually increased her treadmill walking program to three miles, four times a week. In between she enrolled in a step aerobics class and ultimately became one of the best (and certainly the oldest) step aerobics instructors in central Massachusetts. With her exercise program, volunteer work, and studies, her schedule became as crowded as when her children were growing. "After years of wishing I had free time," she confided, "what I found was that I enjoy being active and busy. I was less tired with the new activities than with my golf. In fact, I was energized—physically, intellectually, and spiritually."

It was no wonder that Mary's walk time was so unusual. This was one unusual lady. Her walk time simply reflected what she had trained herself to do over the previous decade: to think, act, and function like a much younger woman. Let me modify that statement: Her training had allowed her to function like a sixty-eight-year-old woman at her personal peak—physically, intellectually, and spiritually. There is no reason to attribute these functions to a younger woman.

Now she was seeking more. The encounter with my laboratory had piqued her curiosity about the potential to use science to push her personal program even further. She booked the appointment with me for follow-up.

Mary's medical history was largely unremarkable. Her only operations had been an emergency appendectomy in her twenties and a cesarean section for the birth of her last child at age thirty. She did not smoke, she drank moderately, and she was of course an avid exerciser. Her physical examination was impressive. Her weight of 117 pounds for her five-foot-four-inch height gave her an excellent Body Mass

Index of 20. Her blood pressure of 120/78 mm Hg was excellent. Her resting heart rate of 62 was excellent for her age and reflected her superb aerobic conditioning. Her strength and flexibility were slightly below what I wanted, and she had evidence of mild osteoarthritis in one knee and both hands. Her laboratory data were fine, including an excellent cholesterol of 180 mg/dl and cholesterol/HDL ratio of 3.5:1. A mammogram, a colonoscopy, and hearing and vision tests, scheduled to get her preventive medical profile up-to-date, were also normal.

After I shared these outstanding results with Mary and complimented her on her positive lifestyle, we got down to work. To address the flexibility and strength issues, Mary would increase her stretching program and begin resistance strength training. I also advised better brands of walking and cross-training shoes to minimize the pounding from her active lifestyle on her knees.

Over the next ten years it was always a pleasure seeing Mary on my patient schedule. True to her word, she maintained her program to forestall becoming "a little old lady." Her aerobic capacity remained largely unchanged, her strength actually improved over 20 percent, and she held a good weight and body fat. Early in our time together she had graduated from night school in library science and now taught high school students how to pursue references for their term papers by surfing the Internet.

At the age of seventy-eight Mary epitomized the results of a personal program to maximize function and slow physiologic aging. I was eager to have my star pupil participate in the Advil Fit over Forty Standards project, and she readily agreed.

Here's how she did:

MARY'S PERSONAL FITNESS PROFILE SCORECARD

The Tests	Mary's Data	Average Data for Her Age and Sex
Fifty-Foot Walk Time	9.0 seconds	8.2–9.5 seconds
Physical Activity Tests	7	2–5
One-Mile Walk Test	16 minutes 43 sec.	20:00–21:48

(continued)

The Tests	Mary's Data	Average Data for Her Age and Sex
Thirty-second Balance Test	6.3 seconds	1.5–2.6 seconds
Sit-and-Reach Flexibility Test	16.8 inches	12.9–16.4 inches
Mind-Body Stress Test	Sometimes experiences stress	Sometimes experiences stress
Upper Body Strength Test	24 reps	18–21 reps
Lower Body Strength Test	23 reps	23–25 reps
Nutritional Habits	18	12–14
Body Fat Tests		
Body Mass Index	20	27
Waist-to-Hip Ratio	0.7	0.8–1.0

As Mary's data reveal, this is not a "little old lady"! Clearly, eight out of her ten test results on the Advil Fit over Forty Standards put her in the above average or excellent categories for her age and sex, while the other two are average. In fact, her overall result is above average for a woman in her fifties and a solid average for a woman in her forties, compared to the other 348 individuals we tested. Not bad for a woman at the ripe "young" age of seventy-eight!

But Mary's physiologic data tell only a small part of the story. She is one of the most defiantly optimistic, fully alive, incorrigibly funny people I have ever met. Mary is one of the people who convinced me to write this book.

Mary's not lucky. But she is fortunate. She is fortunate that she has been smart enough to live her life fully and consciously and choose her habits judiciously. At seventy-eight Mary is more alive than many people in their forties. Not surprisingly, her results are well deserved, in fact almost predictable.

CAN YOU SLOW THE AGING PROCESS?

Yes. Most definitely! In fact, the data from research on slowing physiologic and cognitive processes of aging have become so persuasive that the real question is not *can* you slow the aging process, but *how much*. We have begun to redefine what healthy aging is all about.

PHYSIOLOGIC VERSUS CHRONOLOGICAL AGE

Each of us carries three ages: our chronological age, our physiologic age, and our mind-body, or spiritual, age. Our *chronological age* reflects the number of years we have been on the planet. Our *physiologic age* reflects how well our bodily processes function; this in turn depends largely on how well we have taken care of ourselves and what we have done on a daily basis. Our *mind-body (spiritual) age* reflects our cognitive function and enthusiasm for life. I'll have more to say about this "third" age later in the chapter. But with regard to the first two ages, as Mary's case beautifully illustrates, there can be an enormous disparity between chronological and physiological age.

A general way to look at these ages is depicted below. As this chart

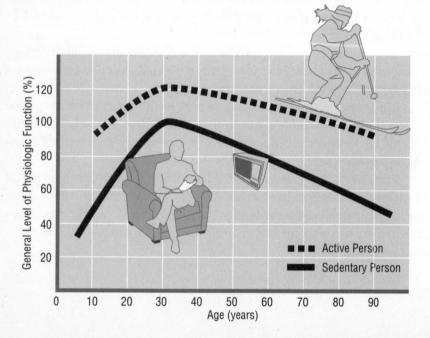

reveals, an active person builds a larger physiologic capacity than an inactive one and experiences more gradual decline. But I think the picture may be even brighter than this illustration indicates. There are huge differences from person to person, and when mental and cognitive functions are factored into the mix, I believe it is possible to carry virtually 100 percent of mind-body fitness well into the seventies and beyond.

The point I am making is a simple one. Our chronological age reflects the date we were born. Our physiologic and mind-body ages reflect the way we choose to live.

How much can we slow the hands of time? We do not know. But if my years as a physician and health and fitness researcher have taught me one thing about this, it is that Mary's accomplishments can become the rule rather than the exception—but only if we put the lessons we have learned to work for us.

LESSONS FROM THE ADVIL FIT OVER FORTY STANDARDS PROJECT

While Mary's results were extraordinary, she was by no means the only exceptional participant in the Advil Fit over Forty Standards project. In each decade and for both sexes we found a handful of people whose results clearly defined the power of daily practices and habits. Of course, we also found plenty of people whose results cried out for improvement. In the final analysis two lessons became abundantly clear. First, even though we studied such areas as cardiovascular fitness, strength, balance, and physical activity separately, in reality they were closely linked to one another. Improvement in one was often translated into improvements in others, conversely, deficits in one often carried over into problems in others. Second, there was a small group of individuals who, through their daily actions, had chosen to lead their lives on a different physical, mental, and spiritual level. These were the people who led physically active, intellectually searching, optimistic lives.

Their experiences and achievements mirror the new insights we are gaining into the science of physiologic and cognitive aging. Using the same components of fitness that are discussed throughout *Fit over Forty*, let's look at how we can use these insights to help us, like Mary and these other high achievers, "stay in the game" for the rest of our lives.

CARDIOVASCULAR FITNESS

Recent studies have altered forever the way we approach cardio-vascular fitness as we grow older. Researchers used to believe that cardiovascular endurance peaked for most people between the ages of twenty and thirty and declined slowly and steadily as they grew older. Now we know that the decline in cardiovascular fitness often observed after the age of forty is probably a result of decreased activity and the societal expectation that as we age, we should become more sedentary. We also know that the phenomenal retention of aerobic capacity that Mary experienced mirrors the experiences of virtually any individual—*provided* that he or she maintains his or her level of physical activity. Remember that Mary had dramatically increased her cardiovascular endurance between the ages of fifty-five and fifty-eight, maintained this high level in the decade between fifty-eight and sixty-eight, and only experienced a 5 percent decline between sixty-eight and seventy-eight. I firmly believe that if her arthritic knee had not slowed her walking pace a bit, she would have maintained a steady cardiovascular capacity for the two decades between fifty-eight and seventy-eight.

Studies by Dr. Robert Bruce and colleagues in Seattle showed that active individuals do experience a slight decline in cardiovascular fitness from their fifties onward, but the rate of decline is less than one third as fast as sedentary individuals! Many other studies that have followed active individuals over long periods have shown similar results. In my own life I have experienced a 10 percent increase in my aerobic capacity in the two decades between twenty-eight and forty-eight.

In my laboratory we have even gone a step further. We have shown that individuals in their fifties, sixties, and seventies can dramatically increase their cardiovascular fitness through a program of structured walking. In one study of volunteers between the ages of seventy and seventy-nine, the average gain in cardiovascular fitness was 15 percent over a twelve-week walking period. If regular physical activity is not the fountain of youth for cardiovascular fitness, it is the next thing to it.

In addition to increasing cardiovascular capacity, regular physical activity significantly reduces the risk of developing heart disease, and it's never too late to achieve this benefit. In one study conducted by Dr. Paffenbarger and his colleagues, even individuals in their sixties who started regular physical activity cut their risk of cardiovascular disease for the rest of their lives. Remember, when you reach the age of sixty-five in the United States, you have a greater than 80 percent chance of living into your eighties, and reducing your risk of heart disease can make those years truly a prize.

STRENGTH

Loss of strength is probably the most underrated health hazard of aging. Fortunately it is possible to prevent this decline entirely. As I have already mentioned, after the age of forty, the areas of cardiovascular fitness and strength grow closer and closer together for every decade that you live. In addition to its interaction with cardiovascular fitness, adequate muscular strength is important for balance, walk speed, and simply navigating the activities of daily living.

From a series of wonderful studies performed by my colleagues at the USDA Human Nutrition Research Center on Aging at Tufts, we have learned that men and women over the age of fifty can experience significant benefits from strength training, including improved strength, balance, and bone mass. Researchers at Boston University recently showed that individuals in their *nineties* achieved significant gains in strength and mobility after a well-constructed strength training program. The final benefit, already discussed, is the preservation or increase in lean muscle tissue that is so vital for lifelong weight management.

Regular strength training stands right next to cardiovascular fitness activity as two pillars of my antiaging program for every person over the age of forty.

PHYSICAL ACTIVITY

In addition to the many benefits discussed in Chapter 5, consistent physical activity is a potent antiaging strategy. I cannot overemphasize the key role of regular physical activity as an antiaging strategy. In fact, in multiple studies, level of physical activity has been more closely linked with physiologic function than any other parameter. I suspect that this is partially due to the strong interaction among physical activity, cardiovascular activity, strength, and functional fitness.

If I had one piece of advice to give people who want to slow or stop the physiologic process of aging, it would be to maintain or increase physical activity throughout their lives. Tragically most people do exactly the opposite. Participation in regular physical activity declines through every decade in life to the point that major studies have documented that less than 10 percent of adults over sixty achieve enough physical activity. We've got to do better in our ability to function. Our health, our very lives depend upon it. So if you skipped over Chapter 5, go back and read it now.

NUTRITION

Poor nutrition is the silent killer of people over the age of forty and a major factor accelerating the aging process. I've already discussed the concepts of sound nutrition that apply to everyone over the age of forty. Let me add several comments about nutrition and aging.

While many people in their forties and fifties battle with weight gain, over the age of sixty, weight *loss* and inadequate calorie intake coupled with unbalanced nutritional practices become the predominant problem. There are two major reasons for this. First, after sixty, we experience a progressive decline in appetite. Since our appetite no longer warns us when to eat, we may inadvertently lose weight and rob our bodies of adequate nutrients, and unwanted weight loss, particularly when associated with any chronic illness or underlying condition, always carries negative health consequences. As we grow older, therefore, we must make a conscious effort to consume adequate calories.

Second, the nutrient composition of our diets tends to deteriorate as we age. In one study the risk of heart attacks in individuals over sixty-five tripled if their blood level of a particular amino acid, homocysteine, became elevated. The major reason for elevated homocysteine? Inadequate consumption of fruits and vegetables and the folate they contain. It's particularly important to monitor the actual composition of your diet in your sixties and beyond as your appetite begins to decline to ensure adequate vitamin and nutrient intake. It is also a reason why I recommend that all my patients over the age of sixty take a daily multivitamin with folate.

One final word: Just as appetite declines with age, so does thirst, making my previous advice about consuming extra water on a daily basis particularly crucial to individuals over the age of sixty.

DENTAL HEALTH

Healthy teeth and gums also play an important part in proper nutrition (not to mention a nice appearance). Eating crunchy fruits and vegetables, for example, becomes more difficult with dental problems. But with good care—twice-a-day brushing and flossing and twice-a-year preventive dental checkups—your teeth should last a lifetime. Avoid foods high in sugar. Not only are they loaded with empty calories, but they are big contributors to tooth decay.

THE HEALTH OF VARIOUS ORGAN SYSTEMS

None of us will live forever, and there is no doubt that physiologic declines do occur over the years. For example, the kidney function of an average seventy-year-old is approximately 50 percent that of an average thirty-year-old, and the incidence of virtually every chronic disease increases with increasing age. But the point of this chapter and in a sense of this entire book is that each of us has vast latitude and tremendous opportunity to forestall physiologic aging through our daily habits and actions. I am not at all convinced that in a perfect world I would want to live forever, but I sure know that I want to be fully alive every moment I inhabit this all-too-imperfect one.

An active lifestyle, proper nutrition, and effective weight management reduce the risk of virtually every chronic disease associated with aging—heart disease, diabetes, cancer, diabetes, osteoarthritis, and hypertension, to name a few. The older we get, the more we associate good health with the absence of disease.

While I believe that good health is much more than this, isn't it comforting to know that the same practices that enhance fitness and function also fight disease?

I also recommend that you schedule regular "preventive" checkups with your physician. Remember, when I first saw Mary, I ordered mammography, colonoscopy, and vision and hearing tests to bring her preventive program up-to-date. Depending on your age, sex, and history, some or all of these tests or others may be appropriate for you. The best advice is to consult with your physician. Keeping you healthy with preventive practices should be the goal of every family doctor in America.

PREVENTIVE MAINTENANCE: ENSURING FUNCTIONAL FITNESS FOR BODY AND MIND

Earlier this year the odometer in my car tripped two hundred thousand miles. I've had "him" (or is it "her"?) for almost ten years and wouldn't trade him for any bright, new shiny model. While I must admit to a certain amount of luck with this car, I've also played a role in his longevity. He's had his oil changed religiously every five thousand miles, and every other item of preventive maintenance has been done consistently and by the book.

Why do we pay more attention to preventive maintenance of our autos than our own health? Perhaps it is because the consequences of failure to do so are obvious and inconvenient. Don't make this mistake when it comes to your health and fitness.

As discussed fully in Chapter 6, both health and function become overriding concerns for all of us over forty. Luckily the decline in function—physical and mental—that we all fear can be reversed, or at least significantly forestalled, through the same lifestyle choices that foster improved cardiovascular fitness, strength, and physical activity. Our research clearly shows that cardiovascular fitness, strength, and level of physical activity all correlate with such critical functional parameters as mobility, balance, and reaction time. And just as there is no reason to accept physical decline, so there is no reason to grow old mentally. In both these areas, like the others just discussed, the maxim "Use it or lose it" again applies.

It seems to me that what sets apart people like Dr. Ted Phillips and Mary and those who excelled in the Advil Fit over Forty Standards tests is that they are explorers. They keep their bodies fit and functional with a conscious commitment to exercise and nutrition. They keep their intellects alive and plastic by seeking new challenges: at age eighty taking up the piano; at seventy-five teaching high school kids how to surf the Internet; at seventy organizing a major new project for a community group. All these individuals have remained calm but adventuresome or, as Eliot says, "still and still moving." We can do the same by following their lead.

EIGHT RULES TO SLOW THE AGING PROCESS

How can we adopt the kinds of practices that allow us to maintain the vigor and youthful spirit and energy we all desire? The answers vary for each of us, of course, but here's a starter list of eight principles I have culled from the most successful patients I have had the privilege to look after.

Rule 1: Don't accept chronological age. *Physiologic* age more accurately reflects who you are and what you do.

Rule 2: Remain physically active.

Rule 3: Be physically strong. Strength retards aging.

Rule 4: Be an explorer—both physically and mentally.

Rule 5: Be your own arbiter of lifestyle habits. Don't accept a sedentary societal expectation.

Rule 6: Be optimistic.

Rule 7: Adopt a consistent preventive maintenance program with your physician.

Rule 8: Be social. Isolation is unhealthy.

FALL

It is nighttime. The chill fall day has given way to the first really cold night; we'll probably have frost tonight. It is a good time to be inside with the people and animals and books that I love. As I grow older, I find more comfort in the ordinary, the sense of order, if you will. Tomorrow will be another clear fall day, and if we're lucky, we'll have a string of another glorious days before a short, intense winter. New England weather can be tricky, but hope springs eternal. (Perhaps the Red Sox will finally win the World Series this year... oh, well.)

Fall in New England truly is, to return to Berryman, "a prize to rouse us toward our fate." For all of us in our forties and beyond, so should this period of our lives be—and it will be—if we make it so.

CHAPTER 15

MAINTAINING FITNESS WHILE COPING WITH SPECIAL HEALTH CONSIDERATIONS

FRANCES

Frances was one of the most beautiful and courageous people I have ever met. She first came to my office one spring morning in the early 1980s at the suggestion of her oncologist, who is one of the new breed of doctors who emphasize total patient care—both body and soul, in addition to all the high tech wizardry readily available in major medical facilities. Three months before, Frances had been diagnosed with breast cancer and undergone a radical mastectomy. A $1\frac{1}{2}$-centimeter cancerous mass had been removed with a node dissection revealing five nodes positive for malignant spread of the tumor. Frances was now facing several rounds of aggressive chemotherapy.

"I have a very clear agenda, Dr. Rippe," she said. "I have a serious disease. I didn't ask for this. I didn't want it. I'm trying not to be mad that I got it. But the bottom line is that I have cancer. Now it seems to me that either I can roll over and start to die now, or I can live my life to the fullest every day for as many days as I have. I've chosen life. Dr. Lancaster says you can help me, and I'd like you to try."

In the early 1980s our knowledge of exercise, nutrition, and mind-body techniques as components of an overall treatment program for cancer was still at a relatively primitive stage, but I resolved to help Frances as much as I could. A walking program was the first order of business. I knew that it would raise her spirits, and some studies were beginning to show that exercise stimulated the immune system, which is so important to fighting off cancer. I also was concerned about her diminished range of motion in her right arm. Prior to her surgery, Frances had been an avid tennis player. But the radical mastectomy had weakened a number of muscles, and the standard exercises prescribed by her surgeon, while okay for the activities of daily living, were inadequate to give her the range of motion she needed to play tennis. I asked an excellent physical therapist to help with this. Since sound nutrition would also be key to Frances's ongoing recovery, we talked about such basics as increasing fruits and vegetables, lowering fat, and maintaining adequate calorie consumption, and I also enlisted the aid of one of our hospital nutritionists.

My final recommendation tapped into Frances's passion for reading. Bernie Siegel's first book *Love, Medicine & Miracles* had just been published, and I urged Frances to read it. Dr. Siegel's book had caused quite a stir with both the public and the medical profession. In it he advocates visualization, guided imagery, and verbalization as components of therapy for cancer. Most important, he emphasizes the power of love and hope. Even though many of my colleagues dismissed Dr. Siegel's theories out of hand (most, it seemed, without reading it), I thought his message was important. Here was a man reminding us of the power of the human spirit and what it meant to be not just a doctor but a *healer*. Dr. Siegel wasn't shunning traditional medicine; rather he was embracing and enhancing it. Far from denouncing standard cancer therapies, he was offering a way to extend them. Most important, he was reminding us of the healing power of hope and love and the obligation every physician assumes to use every tool at his or her disposal and never to abandon a patient even if traditional therapies fail. I believed (and still believe) that it was an important message for Frances to hear, one that we in the medical community too often forget to deliver.

The first three months of chemotherapy, such as those Frances was starting, are always hard. At some point in the future I hope we will be able to harness molecular biology and genetic engineering so that we can develop drugs that attack only cancer cells. For now, unfortunately, we must use drugs designed to take advantage of the fact that cancer cells grow and divide rapidly. As these drugs attack rapidly dividing cancer cells, they also attack other rapidly dividing normal cells, such as those of the gastrointestinal tract, hair follicles, and bone marrow. Destruction of these innocent bystanders leads to unpleasant side effects, such as nausea and vomiting, hair loss, anemia, and infections. A small price to pay for effective chemotherapy—but very disconcerting for all involved—patient, family, and doctors alike. Frances faced these challenges with her customary courage and positive attitude.

When I saw Frances a month after her first round of chemotherapy, she beamed at me when I entered the exam room. The former brunette was now bedecked in auburn curls. "I always wanted to be a redhead." She laughed, flipping back her wig to reveal a totally bald pate. "You guys just speeded the process by giving me God's ultimate haircut!"

Frances had gone through the usual misery of nausea and vomiting and hair loss, but it hadn't dampened her fighting spirit. Her physical therapy was going well, and she had gained enough motion in her right arm to resume tennis. Her appetite was good, and her weight stable.

"Even when my red and white blood cell counts fell," she joked, "the good news was that so did my cholesterol!"

She and her husband had bought a dog and were walking almost every day—sometimes twice a day. She had read Bernie Siegel's book cover to cover and was now visualizing herself cancer-free and keeping a journal. "There's a reason why God gave me this special challenge," she said, "and my job is to figure out why."

Over the next seven years Frances and I and her other doctors and family went through many ups and a few downs. Through it all she taught me the power of hope and the meaning of dignity. When her cancer broke through one type of chemotherapy, she pursued the next, facing a whole new and different round of side effects. She walked on most days, visualized and meditated every day, and drew her family and friends toward her in a way that she never had before her illness.

Seven and a half years after her initial diagnosis, Frances died in her sleep, surrounded by her children and grandchildren and secure in the knowledge that even though she had finally surrendered to her cancer, she had lived those years fully and intentionally: She had chosen life.

Frances had also more than doubled the time that most experts would have predicted for her survival. Lucky? Perhaps, but I find it hard to believe that her optimism, visualization, love for and from her family, walking, and sound nutrition, coupled with the excellent medical care she received from her team of physicians, didn't contribute to her survival.

POSITIVE LIFESTYLE IN CHRONIC ILLNESS AND OTHER SPECIAL CIRCUMSTANCES

By the time we reach our forties, most of us are either in or fast approaching the second half of our lives. In addition, by the time we reach our forties and fifties, all of us know people who have died from acute or chronic illnesses, and many of us will have acquired at least one chronic condition that requires attention and perhaps modification of our lifestyles and habits. In short, by the time we reach our forties, we've had a hefty dose of reality. We know, some of us all too well, that we are not immortal. As one of my friends once said, "Up to the age of forty God takes care of you. After that you'd better be prepared to lend Him (or Her!) a hand."

Although this entire book has focused on the daily decisions and practices each of us can adopt to increase vitality and decrease the likelihood of contracting chronic diseases, the reality, of course, is that at some point we will have to cope with a chronic condition and perhaps a serious illness. The good news is that over the past decade dramatic progress has been made not only in the prevention but also in the treatment of virtually every chronic illness or condition common to people over forty. Through this book I've discussed how daily practices such as exercise, proper nutrition, and mind-body strategies can help you stay fit and lower your risk of chronic disease. In this chapter I want to look at how lifestyle issues can help you cope with and treat such conditions if you already have one. For some conditions, I'll also look at how lifestyle choices can help you control various risk factors, since controlling these is usually as important to treatment as to prevention. The areas we'll look at include heart disease, cancer, diabetes, arthritis, hypertension, other chronic illnesses, and sports injuries. In addition, since the number of women having babies in their forties has more than doubled in the past decade, I'll even talk about the latest lifestyle information related to healthy pregnancy and childbirth.

HEART DISEASE

As a cardiologist I naturally turn my attention first to lifestyle issues related to cardiovascular disease. My professional bias aside, it is also the most logical place to start for two very important reasons: First, despite dramatic reductions in the incidence of coronary heart disease in the United States over the last two decades, it remains by far the number one killer of men and women in the United States—particularly those over forty—and second, we have available by far the most comprehensive information about lifestyle practices and their ability both to reduce risk and to provide helpful therapies for heart disease.

Although we've discussed lifestyle factors in the prevention and treatment of heart disease in a number of previous chapters, this issue is so important that I want to remind you of several key concepts. The primary concept to remember about lifestyle choices in preventing and treating heart disease is that the incidence of heart disease is directly related to a variety of major and minor risk factors. Major risk factors, those with clear-cut and strong relationships to the likelihood of developing heart disease, include elevated blood cholesterol, hypertension, cigarette smoking, and an inactive lifestyle. There are two important facts to remember about these major factors for heart disease. First, each is independently and strongly related to the risk of developing coronary heart disease. If you have any one of these four risk factors, you double your risk of developing heart disease. Second, the risk factors *multiply* one another rather than add to one another. Thus, if you have one major risk factor for heart disease, your risk doubles. With two, your risk quadruples, and so on. The minor risk factors for heart disease, those that increase the risk of heart disease somewhat less than the major risk factors, include diabetes, a positive family history of heart disease (by this I mean a first-degree relative who has suffered heart disease before the age of sixty-five), obesity, and high levels of stress.

By far the most important take-home message about heart disease and its risk factors is that virtually all of them (with the exception of family history and possibly diabetes) are under your control. No one can guarantee that you'll never contract heart disease, but you sure can tilt the odds in your favor—and the way to do that is regular physical activity, low-fat eating, blood pressure control, and avoiding cigarettes.

What if you already have heart disease? Once again, the message is very positive. Your daily decisions related to these same risk factors can dramatically slow (or even to some degree reverse) the process and lower your risk of subsequent problems. Well-controlled research studies have shown that exercise, smoking cessation, cholesterol control, and blood pressure control helps individuals who already have heart disease both lower their risk of subsequent heart problems and improve their quality of life.

Of course, if you already have heart disease, any program of lifestyle modification needs to take place under physician supervision to assure your safety. Unfortunately the medical profession has been slow to embrace such programs. For example, only one third of the millions of individuals who have heart attacks or undergo open heart surgery or coronary angioplasty each year are enrolled in cardiac rehabilitation programs—despite their proven benefit. If you have heart disease, insist that your physician enroll you in such a program. It could save your life.

A last word about positive lifestyle changes and heart disease: Lately we've heard about aggressive lifestyle measures undertaken possibly to "reverse" narrowed coronary arteries. Some of these programs have featured extremely low-fat diets combined with meditation and exercise while others have employed less restrictive diets in combination with powerful cholesterol-lowering drugs and regular exercise.

My view is that such programs can be beneficial and actually result in reversing at least a portion of coronary artery narrowing. The key to all these programs seems to be to drive the total cholesterol and LDL cholesterol to very low levels. A total cholesterol in the 120 to 130 mg/dl range seems to be ideal. Achieving this level through diet alone, however, is very difficult unless you are extremely dedicated, since calories from fat must be held below 10 percent. A more practical approach for most people is a diet containing approximately 20 percent of calories from fat combined with one of the modern cholesterol-lowering drugs. There is no reason for a person who does not already have established heart disease or an elevated cholesterol to lower the fat in his or her diet to below 20 percent of calories.

CANCER

Lifestyle choices are critical not only to preventing cancer in the first place but also to treating it effectively if you already have it. Let me tell you a statistic that I find absolutely staggering. In a survey conducted a few years ago 50 percent of the respondents agreed with the statement that cancer was an "act of God" and that there wasn't anything any of us could do to prevent ourselves from getting cancer. It's appalling that so many people are so misinformed when in reality there's a lot we can do through our lifestyle choices to lower our risk of contracting various cancers and to help us fight them if we do get them.

To start, the American Cancer Society estimates that over 60 percent of cancers have lifestyle factors as major underlying causes. For example, we could eliminate 35 percent of cancers overnight if everyone in the country stopped smoking. Another 15 percent could be eliminated if we all maintained ideal body weights. Another 5 to 10 percent could be eliminated if we reduced unprotected exposure to the ultraviolet rays of the midday sun. Other cancers are clearly related to environmental toxins and exposures, which can be reduced through new legislation or simply better enforcement of laws currently on the books. We've got to stop viewing cancer as beyond our control and take positive steps.

Fortunately we have wonderful new information to guide our daily lifestyle decisions concerning cancer risk. Three major studies— one in over seventeen thousand male college graduates followed for twenty-five years, another in over one hundred thousand female nurses followed for more than a decade, and a third in over ten thousand individuals (men and women) followed for a decade—have shown that regular physical activity reduces the risk of cancers. The main cancers where risk was reduced are those of the colon, breast, and prostate.

How much physical activity is required to lower your risk of these cancers? Surprisingly little. For the previous sedentary person briskly walking as little as a mile a day consistently throughout your life will substantially reduce your risk of cancers. What do I mean by "substantially"? Most studies suggest this level of physical activity will cut your cancer risk in half. How does physical activity lower the risk of cancer? The honest answer is that we don't know with complete certainty, but theories abound. Exercise stimulates the immune system and lowers body fat, both of which may lower cancer risk. Exercise also increases the speed of feces through the gastrointestinal tract, and that may also play a role in reducing the risk of colon cancer.

Many dietary practices are also clearly related to cancer risk. As I've already indicated, I believe the single most important dietary practice we all can adopt to lower our risk of colon cancer is to consume a minimum of five daily servings of fruits and vegetables. Fruits and vegetables appear to lower the risk of colon cancer because of their high fiber content, possibly their antioxidant content, and other substances and chemicals yet to be identified. One word of caution in this area: An increasing number of pills and capsules that claim to carry all the health-promoting substances found in fruits and vegetables are appearing on the market. There isn't a shred of evidence that these work. Don't use them.

High-fat diets (by which I mean the *average* American diet) have been clearly shown to be related to prostate cancer, probably to breast cancer, and possibly to colon cancer. Fats in the diet probably promote cancer growth and development through stimulating excess levels of estrogen and/or testosterone that play a role in the initiation and development of these particular cancers.

Excess alcohol consumption (more than three alcoholic drinks a day) is associated with increased cancers of the gastrointestinal tract, most notably the liver, esophagus, and stomach. Yet another reason to pay attention to the amount of alcohol consumed and not exceed moderate levels.

Even modest amounts of excess weight are also associated with increased risk of cancers in both men and women. In the Nurses' Health Study, the ongoing study of over one hundred thousand middle-aged female nurses, women who were 60 percent over ideal weight for height doubled their risk of cancers. Those women who were morbidly obese (double or more than their desirable weight for their height) increased their risk of cancer by 400 percent!

Of course, cigarette smoking is the number one cause of preventable cancers in the United States. If you smoke a pack of cigarettes a day, you increase your risk of lung cancer by thirty times (an expanded risk of 3,000 percent). Unfortunately smokers also harm the health of others around them. A recent report from the Environmental Protection Agency classified sidestream smoke (the smoke you inhale as an innocent bystander when you are in a room where another person is smoking) as a potent carcinogen. Just one more of hundreds of reasons not to smoke!

Finally, for all of us sun lovers (yes, I certainly am one) there is no such thing as a healthy tan. Exposure to excessive amounts of ultraviolet radiation from the sun, particularly during midday hours, is definitely associated with increased risk of all types of skin cancer. Sunburns are particularly dangerous. In one major study individuals who had experienced more than six episodes of significant sunburning in childhood tripled their risk of skin cancer. Skin cancer is the fastest-growing epidemic of any type of cancer—probably because of ozone depletion. So cover up.

In addition to lowering your risk of developing cancer in the first place, various lifestyle practices can make important contributions to cancer therapy. Regular exercise and sound nutrition are often keys to both physical and spiritual recovery. Mind-body techniques, such as visualization and psychotherapy, can play major roles in cancer recovery. One study by Dr. David Spiegel and colleagues at Stanford University demonstrated that women with metastatic breast cancer doubled their survival times by participating in supportive group therapy.

So what's the bottom line when it comes to cancer? I believe that we've only scratched the surface when it comes to the potential for lifestyle practices and habits to lower our risk of developing cancer or assist in the treatment of established cancer. I don't think the experience I shared with Frances was an isolated case. We're not victims. We can fight back against cancer.

DIABETES

For the past fifty years lifestyle measures have been the cornerstone of diabetes therapy since exercise and sound nutrition have long been used along with insulin as standard treatment. Now current research has further underscored how powerful our daily actions are in preventing and treating this common disease.

Two recent large studies of men and women have shed new light on the prevention of Type II, or adult-onset, diabetes (the type affecting 95 percent of those with this disease). In both these studies regular physical activity significantly reduced the likelihood of developing adult-onset diabetes even if it did not result in weight loss. Maintaining a desirable body weight would further reduce the risk of diabetes.

For individuals who already have established diabetes, regular exercise is one of the mainstays of therapy. Aerobic exercise enhances the muscles' ability to take in sugar and reduces the need for insulin or oral medicines. Of course, regular exercise also is a key to weight management, which is crucial in diabetes, and reduces the risk of heart disease, one of the feared complications of diabetes.

Diet is an important part of diabetes therapy. Using the consensus of important new research, The American Diabetes Association has issued new dietary guidelines recommending more individualization of nutritional management in diabetes. While simple sugars should still be minimized, the new guidelines emphasize the consumption of monounsaturated fats, such as olive oil, in combination with complex carbohydrates to minimize the increase in blood triglycerides. My best advice to you on this issue if you have diabetes is to consult with a hospital-based nutritionist with special expertise in diabetes, who can explain these new guidelines and adapt them to your diet.

One last word on diabetes: The major threat faced by people with diabetes are the complications that often ultimately accompany the disease. Particularly common is damage to the kidneys, nervous system, heart, and eyes. All these complications are based on the damage diabetes wreaks on small blood vessels, which supply these organs. We now have definitive proof that "tight" control of blood sugar throughout the day substantially reduces these complications. If you have diabetes and are not being treated with a regimen that tightly controls your blood sugar, you should be. Consult with a diabetologist to get on a program of medicine and lifestyle practices that will keep your blood sugar under tight control. It could save your life.

ARTHRITIS

Arthritis is one of the most common chronic conditions for people over forty. One out of every eight people in the United States has arthritis. One out of every four people over the age of fifty suffers from the condition, and over 50 percent of individuals over the age of 65 have significant arthritis in at least one joint. Arthritis is so common with advancing age that I can remember one of my medical school teachers stating that we'll all get arthritis if we're lucky enough to live long enough.

While arthritis is rarely life-threatening, it can be extremely debilitating. In individuals over sixty, arthritis accounts for as many days in bed each year as does heart disease. But over the past ten years we have experienced a dramatic change in our thinking about the management of arthritis. When I was in medical school twenty years ago, the dogma was that those with arthritis should minimize activity, particularly during flare-ups. Now we know that just the opposite is true. Regular physical activity, in combination with proper anti-inflammatory therapy, is just what the doctor ordered (at least this doctor), particularly for the treatment of osteoarthritis, the most common form. Physical activity is effective because the motions it uses are crucial to the healthy movement of fluid and chemicals through the diseased joint or joints.

Of course, you should consult with your personal physician or arthritis specialist if you have this condition and want to be more physically active, but you have a number of excellent options. Water exercise, such as swimming, water walking, or water aerobics, represents an excellent choice for individuals with arthritis since the water supports most of your weight and minimizes excessive impact on joints. Walking programs are also excellent for people with arthritis—even arthritis of the weight-bearing joints of the hip and knee—but be sure to wear appropriate shoes.

Although many claims for nutritional therapies (such as shark cartilage) have been made for arthritis, I am not convinced that any of them offer any proven benefit. Of course, maintaining proper weight is very important since extra weight increases impact on the joints. Otherwise all the principles of sound human nutrition discussed throughout this book apply equally to people with arthritis.

People used to say that despite all the proven benefits of regular physical activity, the one danger to which regular exercisers exposed themselves was the eventual and inevitable onset of arthritis caused by overuse of the joints, particularly the weight-bearing ones. Now we have excellent evidence that this is not true, that just the opposite is true. A long-term study of distance runners in California showed that they had less arthritis and less overall disability than age-matched controls who were sedentary. It turns out that one of the most dangerous things you can do to your joints is not use them.

OSTEOPOROSIS

Osteoporosis, or the progressive loss of bone density, is one of the most common conditions for individuals over the age of forty and the most common disorder of the bones we all confront. While we tend to associate osteoporosis with women, particularly with postmenopausal women, it is also a serious problem in men and the underlying cause of many bone fractures for individuals of both sexes.

Part of the problem we have in confronting osteoporosis is that we make the mistake of thinking that our bones are these solid, inert objects that never change. Nothing could be further from the truth. Our bones are one of the most dynamic, constantly changing organs in the body. Throughout our lives we go through constant cycles of bone growth, dissolution, remodeling and repair. While most of us will achieve our peak bone mass between the ages of thirty to thirty-five and begin a gradual bone loss after this, there is no reason why we can't maintain strong healthy bones throughout our lifetimes.

Whether we are working to prevent or combat osteoporosis there are three issues that contribute to the health of our bones; physical activity, proper nutrition, and, in some postmenopausal women, hormonal replacement. When it comes to our bones, the maxim "Use it or lose it" clearly applies. Regular weight-bearing exercise, such as walking or jogging, is a crucial element of building and maintaining bone mass and strength. Strength training is important as well. In one study of women in their seventies who performed regular strength training exercises for a year, increases in bone strength and density, muscle strength, and balance were achieved. Inactivity is hazardous to your bones.

One caution, however: If you already have osteoporosis, you should work with your physician to ensure that your activity program is safe for you. You may need to make certain modifications to your activities and to be sure too that you have equipment (such as well-padded shoes designed to absorb impact) that protects you.

In addition to exercise, we must consume adequate amounts of calcium. The National Institutes of Health recommend 1,000 mg of calcium a day for women with adequate estrogen levels and for all men over forty. For postmenopausal women who are not taking estrogen replacements the recommendation increases to 1,500 mg of calcium a day. It is very easy to get adequate calcium in our diets, yet 80 percent of individuals over forty do not consume enough on a daily basis. Remember that low-fat dairy products and green leafy vegetables are good sources of calcium. Calcium supplements in the form of calcium carbonate and calcium citrate are available in many products; there is some evidence that calcium citrate (the form added to some orange juices, for example) may be more available to the body than calcium carbonates.

For postmenopausal women, there is convincing evidence that estrogen replacement slows osteoporosis and dramatically reduces the risk of heart disease. The negative side of estrogen replacement is the slight increased risk of breast and uterine cancers. In my opinion, for most postmenopausal women the clear benefits of estrogen replacement outweigh the small risks. However, since this is a highly individualized decision, my best advice to you is to consult with your personal physician if you are a postmenopausal woman.

HYPERTENSION

Hypertension is one of the most common chronic conditions for men and women over the age of forty. There are sixty million adults with hypertension in the United States. One out of every three individuals over forty suffers from this condition. While there is some debate over what blood pressure constitutes hypertension, here are the measurements I use. For diastolic blood pressure (the bottom number) any pressure between 90 and 104 mm Hg is mild hypertension, between 105 and 114 mg Hg is moderate hypertension, and above 115 mm Hg is severe hypertension. For systolic blood pressure (the top number) any reading between 140 and 159 mm Hg is borderline systolic hypertension while any number above 160 mm Hg is definite systolic hypertension.

The reason we care so much about hypertension is that it is a silent killer. Hypertension is a major risk factor for heart disease and the leading cause of stroke in the United States. Fortunately we have many excellent therapies available to prevent or treat hypertension. The lifestyle prevention and/or treatment of hypertension rests on four pillars: regular physical activity, weight management, sodium restriction, and stress reduction.

Regular moderate-intensity aerobic exercise has been consistently shown to lower blood pressure—in individuals with mild to moderate hypertension and even in those with normal blood pressure. Decreases of 6 to 10 mm Hg in both systolic and diastolic blood pressure are common. These effects occur independent of the weight loss and weight management benefits of regular aerobic activity.

Although aerobic exercise can be very helpful, people with hypertension should be very cautious about strength training because lifting weights (free weights or machine) can cause blood pressure to skyrocket. And lifting heavy weights is absolutely forbidden. So before even considering any strength training, discuss what's appropriate for your condition with your physician. I, for example, allow my patients with mild hypertension to participate in high-repetition, low-weight strength training exercises for muscle toning once their blood pressure is under control.

Weight loss and weight management are also critically important to blood pressure control. Decreases of 1 to 2 mm Hg in both systolic and diastolic blood pressure for every pound lost reliably occur in overweight individuals with hypertension. Often for my sedentary, slightly overweight patients with mild hypertension, regular exercise and weight loss are all that is necessary for complete blood pressure control. Remember, regular aerobic exercise combined with a proper low-fat diet is the recipe for successful weight loss, and in addition, both independently lower the risk of heart disease.

Sodium restriction is probably a good health-promoting measure for all of us and absolutely essential for people with even mild hypertension. For some reason buried deep in our ancestral gene pool, human beings have an excessive craving for salt. We eat salt-laden processed foods, and salty snacks, and we salt our food—often even before tasting it. All told, the average American adult consumes six to nine grams of salt a day, two to three times the three grams recommended by the American Heart Association. (Three grams is about half a teaspoon.)

The reason that salt consumption is bad for people with hypertension is that it causes them to retain water, and this in turn elevates blood pressure. In over 95 percent of individuals with hypertension, we never establish a specific cause for the condition, but we think that the problem resides in poor salt handling by the kidney.

Stress reduction has been reliably demonstrated to lower blood pressure in individuals who have underlying anxiety. The heart rate biofeedback technique I described in Chapter 9 is particularly effective for lowering blood pressure.

While all these lifestyle modalities can be extremely helpful in controlling blood pressure, they should be undertaken only in conjunction with your physician. In some instances, particularly in moderate to severe hypertension, drug therapy will be required in addition to these lifestyle measures for complete blood pressure control. There are some wonderful new agents on the market, such as long-acting calcium blockers and ACE inhibitors, that help control blood pressure with minimal or no side effects.

OTHER CHRONIC ILLNESSES

Lung diseases

I sometimes like to kid my colleagues who are pulmonary specialists that the only reason for the lungs is to supply oxygen to the blood so that the heart can do its job. They fire back that the heart exists only to pump blood through the lungs. Obviously the heart and lungs work together as a unit that is vital to every process of living.

Whether you already have lung disease or want to prevent it, the most important lifestyle factor related to lung disease is avoiding cigarette smoking. While cigarette smoking harms every organ, it is particularly hazardous to the lungs, where it leads to dramatic increases in the incidence of lung cancer and emphysema (also called chronic obstructive pulmonary disease or COPD). The best single health decision any cigarette smoker will ever make, for himself or herself as well as for his or her loved ones is to stop. Of course, it is hard to stop smoking. Cigarettes are terribly addicting—some believe even more addicting than heroin—but it is vital to your health to stop smoking, so you must keep trying. It takes average smokers six to ten attempts at stopping before they finally succeed, but millions have stopped this deadly habit for good.

Although recent studies have shown that the nutritional practice of eating at least two fish meals a week may lower the incidence of COPD in cigarette smokers, don't use this finding as an excuse. The best thing any cigarette smoker can do to solve this problem is still to stop smoking.

Regular exercise is probably more beneficial to the cardiovascular system than to the pulmonary system in terms of building increased capacity. For reasons that no one fully understands, we have much more excess capacity in our lungs than our cardiovascular system at birth. Nonetheless, regular exercise does expand lung capacity and strengthen respiratory muscles. Both these benefits are particularly important for individuals with emphysema, a reason why walking exercise is a standard part of pulmonary rehabilitation programs.

Regular aerobic exercise is also very beneficial for people with asthma, yet many of these individuals don't seize this benefit from fear that exercise may make their asthma worse. With modern asthma medicines this fear is largely unfounded, although if you have asthma, your exercise program should be done in conjunction with your asthma doctor.

Gastrointestinal bleeding

Gastrointestinal bleeding is a major problem, particularly for individuals over the age of sixty for whom it represents the fifth leading cause of hospitalization. A recent study provided another strong reason for regular exercise: to lower the risk of gastrointestinal disease. In this study, those over the age of sixty who engaged in regular aerobic exercise cut their risk of gastrointestinal bleeding from all causes in half. The reason that regular aerobic exercise reduces the risk of gastrointestinal bleeding is probably that it improves blood flow to all the organs of the GI tract.

Anxiety and depression

Numerous lifestyle-related choices can play important roles in preventing or treating anxiety and depression. Certainly regular exercise has been demonstrated to lower both acute and chronic anxiety. Similar benefits have been observed for exercise in situational and chronic depression.

In my experience, many people don't even recognize that they may be suffering from anxiety or depression. Over 80 percent of individuals who come to me complaining of fatigue are anxious or depressed or both. If I can convince them to start and maintain regular exercise programs, the symptoms almost invariably evaporate.

A word of warning: Extremely high levels of exercise (such as training for a marathon or a triathlon) can actually cause anxiety and depression. These feelings are part of the overtraining syndrome in this situation, and the cure is *less* exercise rather than more.

COLDS AND FLU

What do lifestyle issues have to do with infectious disease, such as colds and flu? The answer is "Plenty!" As I've already discussed in Chapter 9, studies have linked stress to susceptibility to the common cold. In addition, there is at least some evidence to suggest that regular exercisers suffer from fewer colds.

The most convincing theory on why regular exercisers may suffer fewer colds is that your body temperature rises slightly when you exercise. The body may interpret this as the beginning of a viral illness and cause the white blood cells—the main infection fighters in the body—to go on alert. This in turn may kill off any viruses before they are able to infect you and cause a cold. While the evidence supporting this theory is not complete, it nonetheless represents an attractive hypothesis for the common experience that many exercisers have that they seem to come down with fewer colds.

The most common question that patients ask me concerning exercise and infectious disease is whether or not they can exercise with colds. The answer to that is yes and no. For most people, exercising with a cold represents no danger. However, if you have a high fever, certainly one above 101°F, I would advise against exercise until your fever goes down. Women who are pregnant should not exercise if they have a cold and fever above 100°F.

There are a few rare instances where a virus may be made worse by exercising, but these are extremely unusual. My best advice to you is to follow common sense and let your symptoms be your guide. If you feel uncomfortable when you begin to exercise with a cold, by all means, stop. Conversely, if the exercise feels comfortable, there is no reason not to continue.

PREGNANCY

Lifestyle issues related to pregnancy are increasingly relevant to women in their forties since in the past decade the number of women over forty in the United States who are having children has more than doubled. Happily we have some wonderful news about pregnancy in general and lifestyle factors related to pregnancy for these women.

First, major advances in genetic screening and obstetrical practice have dramatically improved the outcome of pregnancy in "older" mothers. With good obstetrical practice and proper screening techniques 994 out of 1,000 pregnancies for women in their forties will result in healthy babies. Secondly, there are multiple lifestyle decisions and practices that can enhance their pregnancies.

Regular aerobic exercise has been shown to be safe for both mother and fetus. There are some restrictions and guidelines, of course, and an exercise program should always be undertaken with the guidance and consent of your obstetrician. Some excellent books and videotapes on exercise during pregnancy are commercially available, as is a good set of materials from the American College of Obstetrics and Gynecology. Ask your ob/gyn about such resources.

The nutritional practices I've described elsewhere in this book are absolutely appropriate during pregnancy. Sound nutrition is particularly important for the pregnant woman, who now must remember that she is eating for two.

There are two additional nutritional practices essential for pregnant women in their forties. First, every pregnant woman should be consuming at least 400 mcg of folate every day. The easiest way to obtain this is to take a daily "pregnancy" vitamin. This practice virtually eliminates the possibility of congenital defects of the nervous system in the fetus. Second, all pregnant women should avoid excessive intake of vitamin A during pregnancy. Intakes above 10,000 IU of vitamin A have been associated with birth defects. Read the label on any vitamin you take, and don't exceed 4,000 to 5,000 IU per day. You should also avoid eating large amounts of liver during pregnancy since this organ meat is loaded with vitamin A. It is important to emphasize that beta-carotene (a precursor of vitamin A) is acceptable; it's just vitamin A itself that is not.

INJURY REHABILITATION

Many of the practices I've described throughout this book are designed to reduce your risk of injury—both during physical activity and throughout all your activities of daily living. An inactive lifestyle is an invitation to injury since inactive muscles and tendons become weak and stiff.

Nonetheless, it is almost impossible to go through life without some injuries, and when the inevitable happens, it's encouraging to know that we have learned a great deal about injury prevention and rehabilitation.

If you suffer a mild sprain or strain to a muscle or joint, I recommend RICE—rest, ice, compression, and elevation—and that you use common sense about returning to exercise. Anything more severe should receive prompt medical attention.

If you do experience a more severe injury, the good news is that modern sports medicine techniques can fix almost any injury and that exercise routines can be adapted or modified to respond to it. In addition, modern exercise equipment offers the safest and most comfortable range of options ever available to reduce the likelihood of injury and, if one occurs, to help treat it. But to take advantage of these benefits, you must take the need for injury rehabilitation seriously. If you've had a severe injury or a nagging injury that does not get better, you may need to see a sports medicine specialist and a physical therapist about appropriate treatment and rehabilitation exercise. Then follow through.

The keys to avoiding chronic injury are proper technique, proper equipment, and common sense. Most of the people I see who have chronic injuries have violated one of these three cardinal precepts.

SPECIAL CONSIDERATIONS, SPECIAL OPPORTUNITIES

A few years ago I was privileged to participate in an expert panel convened by the Centers for Disease Control and the American College of Sports Medicine to offer public health guidelines for exercise. When we issued our final report, we tried to offer commonsense guidance that every adult could follow. In addition, we made special mention that individuals with chronic conditions were at particular risk for the diseases of inactivity and had much to gain from simple daily lifestyle decisions.

I still strongly subscribe to this belief. When we're in our forties and beyond, we've entered a special time of our lives. While more and more of us will contract chronic conditions as we age, I view this not as our special problem but as our incredible opportunity to use our daily habits to heal ourselves.

CHAPTER 16

PEACE AND PROSPERITY: SUSTAINING A NEW VISION OF FITNESS

THE JOURNEY

As promised, this whole book has been about a journey, one toward personal peace. In the first chapter I asked you to take my hand and walk across the bridge that connects the land of the dead to the land of the living, the land populated by people leading their lives every day to the fullest. I asked you to take some tests based on the Advil Fit over Forty Standards, the first ever established for men and women over forty, to establish the starting point of the journey. Then one by one we explored the sites ranging from cardiovascular fitness and mind-body interactions to nutrition and weight management. In this chapter I want to review the highlights of our trip and offer you the ten key actions that each of us can take in our daily life to achieve personal peace.

A TEN-POINT PEACE PLAN

Over the years I've had the privilege of helping thousands of people down the road to better health and fitness. I've seen many people succeed beyond their wildest dreams, and regrettably, I've also seen some fail. Through all this I've learned one important fact: The people who succeed focus on simple changes with clear plans. The people who falter don't fail because of some cosmic or complex issue; they usually stumble because they make change too complicated. With this in mind, I offer you the following Ten-Point Peace Plan for improving your health and fitness.

Point 1: Walk

That's right, just walk! Aerobic conditioning is the cornerstone of every health and fitness program. It is the one thing I know that will always benefit patients and that they will enjoy. And when it comes to aerobic conditioning, for 95 percent of us, we're talking about walking.

My laboratory has been the leading research institute for walking information for the past decade. During this period my enthusiasm for walking has grown deeper and deeper. If I could get every adult in the United States (and around the world, for that matter) to take a daily twenty- to thirty-minute walk, I would be willing to retire and consider my major goal accomplished: to do the most I could to improve the health of as many people as possible.

In Chapter 3 I gave you the One-Mile Walk Test to determine your cardiovascular fitness. If you haven't already taken it, I urge you to do so for two reasons: First, it will give you an excellent estimate of your cardiovascular fitness; second, it will show you how enjoyable walking is and what a great workout you can get through this simple activity.

In Chapter 8, I also supplied you with some easy walking workouts for health and fitness, but I can simplify this even further with a story and one piece of advice. Former President Harry Truman was famous for his evening constitutionals. Once a huffing Secret Service agent trying to keep up with the president asked, "How should I walk?" To which President Truman responded with characteristic bluntness, "Walk as though you had somewhere to go!" If you walk twenty to thirty minutes every day at a pace "as though you had somewhere to go," you will accomplish one of the most important health and fitness tasks anyone can ever do—and have a great time doing it.

Point 2: Mind your mind

Remember that there are multiple and profound connections between mind and body. Peace with your physical body without spiritual peace is no peace at all. The techniques to utilize simple mind-body techniques to stimulate both physical and spiritual fitness are very accessible. We just need to use them.

View your exercise session as a time to stimulate and heal your body and mind. Concentrate on your breathing; visualize and focus during your warm-up, exercise session, and cooldown. Adopt a type of exercise that stimulates both mind and body, such as yoga or tai chi. Or just use mind-body techniques such as the Relaxation Response or visualization to enhance activity sessions and turn them into mind-body respites and refreshers.

Point 3: Listen to your heart

The key to stress reduction is to live fully and consciously in the here and now. Regretting the past or fearing the future will fill our lives with negative stress.

One of the most powerful ways to inhabit the here and now is to listen to your body rhythms. In Chapter 9 I describe how a simple ten-minute daily session of monitoring your heartbeat can lead to substantial stress reduction. It sounds almost too good to be true, yet I've seen it work over and over again. Who doesn't have ten minutes each day to lower his or her stress level?

Point 4: Be strong

There's no reason why we have to become weak as we grow older, and getting weaker undermines our health. Weak muscles lead to injuries, increased body fat, discomfort, constricted lifestyles, and ultimately, for far too many individuals, the end of independent living. We've got to recognize strong muscles for what they really are, one of the keys to lifelong healthy, active, independent living. Once you've established a regular walking (or other physical activity) program, the next step is to incorporate two or three twenty-minute strength training sessions into your weekly routine.

Point 5: Stay flexible

Here's the easiest one yet! By walking or, even better yet, by combining walking with regular strength training, you're going to keep your muscles healthy, and healthy muscles are also flexible.

But why not go the next step? By including five minutes of light stretching both before and after activity as part of your warm-up and cooldown, you will improve your flexibility. Even on days when you do not exercise, a light stretching program, such as the one I describe in Chapter 11, can keep your joints and muscles limber and ready and able to meet the challenge of daily living.

Point 6: Use it or lose it

Many people don't realize that our ability to function at our best, whether physically or mentally, is based on the accumulation of effects of our daily habits. People who remain active and vibrant have chosen to use all their abilities and faculties to their fullest potentials. So the best rule each of us can adopt to function at our fullest is to "use it" or else we'll invariably "lose it."

Use your muscles. Exercise for your heart's benefit. Adopt new hobbies. Learn to play a musical instrument. Make a personal commitment not to go quietly into the night.

Point 7: Become an activist

Physical activity saves lives. It is as simple as that. Opportunities to be physically active abound in our lives; we simply have to seize them.

Each of us should try to find ways of accumulating at least thirty minutes of moderate intensity physical activity on most, if not all, days. Of course, if you adopt the walking program I outline in Point 2, you are home free. But don't overlook the many other easy opportunities we have to be more active every day. Do the lawn or housework. Take the stairs, not the elevator. Park and walk. These all count and can easily add up to thirty minutes a day.

Remember, an active lifestyle is a healthy lifestyle.

Point 8: Find peace with food

As discussed in Chapter 12, simple nutritional practices can make an enormous difference in your energy level and well-being and can actually save your life.

While I've outlined a number of these simple alterations in our daily diets, to simplify it even further, I think the single most important practice to adopt is to eat more fruits and vegetables. If we all ate five servings of fruits and vegetables on a daily basis, we would lower the risk of heart disease and cancer and make enormous strides toward ending the epidemic of obesity that threatens our health.

Point 9: Find a healthy weight

Of course, weight management is difficult, but it is not impossible. And it is an issue that over 50 percent of us struggle with on a daily basis. We need to establish a framework that is both medically correct yet reasonable, as I discuss in Chapter 13. Here are two key concepts for healthy weight: First, recognize that weight is a health issue; second, find your own personal healthy weight.

So how does each of us establish a "healthy" weight? I suggest following this straightforward three-step process:

1. Prevent further weight gain. Because at any weight above desirable weight health risks increase with *further* weight gain, the first priority should be to prevent further weight gain.
2. Try to lose ten to fifteen pounds and keep them off. Even if you've gained forty or fifty pounds over your middle years, studies have shown that the risks of weight-related chronic diseases decline significantly for people who lose ten to fifteen pounds and keep them off for at least two years.
3. Find a healthy weight you can maintain for a lifetime. Once you have accomplished Steps 1 and 2, you're in a position to move toward further weight loss and establishment of a healthy, stable weight. The key is to recognize weight control as a lifelong issue for most of us and to adopt the lifelong strategies of increased activity and conscious low-fat eating.

Point 10: Act your (physiologic and spiritual) age

All of us carry three ages: our chronological age (how many years we've been on the planet), our physiologic age (how old our body processes and organ functions are), and our spiritual age (how youthful and plastic our mental processes and perspectives are). Don't get caught in the trap of feeling that the only age that matters is the chronological one. We all know people who look, feel, and function at levels far younger than their chronological ages. Their secret: They have chosen to function at their physiologic and spiritual age—and so can you.

A NEW VISION OF FITNESS

In the late 1980s millions of us saw an enjoyable movie called *Field of Dreams* that presents a story that I think has wonderful implications for health and fitness. Just in case you missed it, allow me to recount the story briefly. It's about an Iowa farmer in his late thirties (of course, he'd be in his mid-forties by now) who starts hearing a voice as he's out working his cornfields. The voice is saying, "If you build it, he will come."

After a great deal of thought the farmer decides that the voice is telling him to cut down his corn crop and build a baseball field. He does this, then figures out what the voice means when it also tells him to "Ease his pain" and "Go the distance" and acts on those instructions. Sure enough, eventually a lot of former baseball greats and important people from the farmer's past start arriving to play baseball on the field. The event changes the farmer's life and that of his family forever and for the better.

Now what does this have to do with health and fitness? Let me explain. I believe that each of us builds the life we lead and the health and happiness we enjoy one day at a time through our daily habits and actions. If we are careful and adopt the simple measures I've discussed throughout this book—if we "build" these bridges—we can achieve higher levels of physical and spiritual well-being than we ever dreamed possible. In a sense, we and only we hold the power to "ease our pain," if we are willing to "go the distance" to live each day fully and consciously.

A PERSONAL JOURNEY

Early in this book I introduced you to a young doctor in his early thirties who thought he knew more than he really did—both in his own health and fitness program and for his patients. As you know, I was that physician. Fortunately over the years I have taken a wonderful journey where I've learned a lot—from patients, from my own health and fitness program, from extensive research in my laboratory and others around the world.

It's been an intensely personal journey. I am not just writing about health and fitness over the age of forty; I'm also living it. At the age of forty-eight I can honestly say that I feel more genuinely happy and fit than I've ever felt in my life.

Nothing in this book is abstract. It's based on putting the lessons I've learned to work with patients in their lives and in my own life. I don't run forty miles a week anymore. My program is now a walk-run combination. I strength train and stretch. The mind-body and stress reduction techniques described in this book are wonderful respites in my very crowded life. I'm slowly coming to peace with food, and my weight has been stable for the past decade.

In the final analysis we all face the same challenges and wonderful complexities and even the sadness of life. I don't think most people over forty want to turn the clock back. I know I don't.

The world is more complicated, and anyone who offers a simple solution doesn't recognize that one of the joys of being over the age of forty is to see some things in all their complexity and understand them for the first time.

But some things *are* simple—at least relatively so. And the simple truth for most of us is that we're trying to do the best we can to live fully, happily and meaningfully. One of the best ways to approach this important, but often elusive, goal is to pay more attention to our daily habits and practices, which can make an enormous difference in our spiritual and physical health and fitness. That is the most direct path for most of us to personal peace and prosperity. And isn't finding peace and prosperity what it's all about?

APPENDICES

FIT OVER FORTY PERSONAL FITNESS
PROFILE SCORECARD

In the column headed "Your Data" record your results on the Fit over Forty tests. In the column headed "Average Data for Your Age and Sex" record the appropriate figures from the Advil Fit over Forty Standards for each test in Chapter 3. Use the final column, headed "Your Goals," as you plan your fitness program, using the information in Chapter 4.

THE TESTS	YOUR DATA	AVERAGE DATA FOR YOUR AGE AND SEX	YOUR GOALS
1. Fifty-Foot Walk Test for Mobility			
2. Physical Activity Test			
3. One-Mile Walk Test for Cardio-vascular Fitness			
4. Thirty-Second Balance Test			
5. Sit-and-Reach Flexibility Test			
6. Mind-Body Stress Reduction Test			
7. Upper Body Strength Test			
8. Lower Body Strength Test			
9. Nutritional Habits Test			
10. Body Fat Tests: Body Mass Index			
Hip-to-Waist Ratio			

SEVEN-DAY MENU PLANS

1,200-CALORIE MEAL PLAN MENUS

Exchanges:

4 Meat	3 Fruit
4 Starch/Bread	3 Fat
3 Vegetable	2 Milk
Open calories: 80	

Day 1

Breakfast

$^1/_3$ cantaloupe
2 slices reduced calorie whole-wheat toast (or 1 slice regular whole-
  wheat) with 2 teaspoons all-fruit spread
1 cup skim or 1 percent milk*
Coffee or tea

Lunch

1-ounce pita (4") or $^1/_2$ 6" pita stuffed with mix of 1 ounce 95% fat-
  free lunch meat, $^1/_4$ cup nonfat cottage cheese, chopped tomatoes, lettuce, sprouts, grated carrots, seasoned with 1
  tablespoon nonfat Italian salad dressing
1 small apple or $^1/_2$ cup applesauce
Noncaloric drink

Snack

2–3 cups air-popped plain popcorn (if you like, season with
  butter-flavored cooking spray and nonfat butter sprinkles)

Dinner

3 ounces fillet of grilled or baked fish
Small (3 ounces) baked potato with 1 tablespoon nonfat sour cream
  or yogurt
$^1/_2$ cup steamed broccoli with lemon-pepper seasoning
1 cup mixed green salad with 1 tablespoon nonfat dressing
$^1/_2$ cup sliced peaches and berries

Open calories: Add a tablespoon of reduced-calorie whipped
dessert topping to your dinner peaches and berries or upgrade your
baked potato to medium size (6 ounces).

*Unless otherwise specified in the menus, milk is always skim or 1 percent. If you use 2 per-
cent or whole milk, add a fat exchange.

Day 2

Breakfast

$\frac{1}{2}$ cup orange or grapefruit juice
$\frac{1}{2}$ cup dry cereal (shredded wheat, oat circles, etc.) with $\frac{1}{2}$ cup milk
1 slice wheat toast with 1 teaspoon fruit spread
Coffee or tea

Lunch

Tuna salad sandwich: 2 slices reduced-calorie wheat or rye bread, $\frac{1}{4}$ cup water-packed tuna mixed with chopped celery, dill-pickle relish, and $\frac{1}{2}$ tablespoon reduced calorie mayonnaise
$\frac{1}{2}$ cup carrot sticks
1 small apple
Noncaloric drink

Snack

Fruit whip: Blend 1 cup strawberries or $\frac{1}{2}$ banana (4.5") with $\frac{1}{2}$ cup nonfat yogurt

Dinner

3 ounces grilled or baked chicken (skinless)
1 cup green salad with nonfat, reduced-calorie dressing
1 cup summer squash medley (sauté or roast a combination of yellow squash, zucchini, green pepper, onion, garlic in 1 teaspoon olive oil)

Open calories: Add a 1-ounce roll to dinner.

Day 3

Breakfast

Orange or half a banana
½ cup oatmeal
1 cup milk
Coffee or tea

Lunch

Salad bar: 2 cups mixed vegetable salad with 1 ounce lean meat or
¼ cup low-fat cottage cheese, 1 tablespoon garbanzo beans, 1
tablespoon reduced calorie or nonfat salad dressing
6 saltine or reduced-calorie Ritz crackers
½ cup fresh fruit from salad bar (pineapple, kiwi, apple or 1 cup
strawberries, melon)
Noncaloric drink

Snack

2 rice cakes with 1 tablespoon peanut butter

Dinner

3 ounces boneless pork tenderloin medallions baked with caraway
seeds and 1 cup slivered red or green cabbage (or ½ cup sauerkraut*)
½ cup stewed apple slices with cinnamon (no sugar added)
½ cup mashed potatoes (whipped with a little skim milk and butter sprinkles)
½ cup frozen nonfat yogurt

Open calories: Increase breakfast oatmeal to 1 cup or have an apple
for another snack.

*high in salt

Day Four

Breakfast

$\frac{1}{2}$ grapefruit
1 bagel with 1 tablespoon reduced-fat cream cheese
1 cup milk

Lunch

1 tomato stuffed with 2 ounces chicken salad prepared with chopped celery, dill-pickle chunks, and $\frac{1}{2}$ tablespoon reduced fat mayonnaise or nonfat Italian dressing
$\frac{1}{2}$ cup celery and carrot sticks
$\frac{1}{4}$ cup raisins
Noncaloric drink

Snacks

2 apricots or plums
1 cup milk or nonfat cocoa

Dinner

1 cup spaghetti with low-fat meat sauce (made with low-fat ground turkey, 2-ounce serving)
1 cup mixed vegetable green salad with nonfat dressing
Noncaloric drink

Open calories: 1 tablespoon grated Parmesan cheese to top the spaghetti or 1-ounce hard roll with dinner.

Day Five

Breakfast

⅓ melon or 1¼ cups watermelon
¾ cup cornflakes or other flake cereal
1 cup milk
Coffee or tea

Lunch

Fast food: 6-inch turkey sub on whole-wheat roll (2 ounces turkey, lettuce, tomato, green pepper, sweet pickled peppers, onion, mustard, splash of oil and vinegar)
1 small apple or orange
Noncaloric drink

Snack

1 cup milk shake made with sugar-free mix

Dinner

Shrimp creole *over ½ cup brown rice (2 ounces shrimp)
Steamed broccoli or carrots
1 cup mixed green salad with 1 tablespoon nonfat dressing
1 cup strawberries
Noncaloric beverage

Open calories: Add a bread exchange or another ½ cup rice with dinner or 1 exchange of pretzels for a snack.

Busy today? Substitute a low-fat/low-calorie frozen dinner with similar ingredients such as those made by Healthy Choice or Lean Cuisine.

*A basic creole sauce is composed of chopped tomatoes, green peppers, and onions sautéed with a bay leaf in a little olive oil.

Day Six

Breakfast

$1/2$ cup orange juice
Scrambled eggs (1 yolk, 2 whites, 1 teaspoon margarine)
1 slice whole-wheat toast (or 2 slices reduced-calorie whole-wheat)
    with 1 teaspoon jelly
Coffee or tea

Lunch

1 cup plain nonfat yogurt mixed with $1/2$ cup fresh fruit (peaches,
    apricots, berries)
1 ounce baked (no-fat) tortilla chips
Noncaloric drink

Snack

1 small apple

Dinner

3 ounces chicken piccata with $1/2$ cup pasta
$1/2$ cup green beans
1 cup salad medley (chunked tomato, cucumber, and carrot
    dressed with balsamic vinegar and dillweed)
$1/2$ cup sugar-free pudding or low-fat (2%) ice cream

Open calories: Add 4 Ry-Krisp crackers as a snack.

Day Seven

Breakfast

$\frac{1}{2}$ cup tomato or orange juice
1 English muffin with 1 teaspoon margarine or fruit spread (or 4
   pancakes [4"] with reduced-calorie syrup using open calories)
1 cup milk or coffee-flavored nonfat yogurt
Coffee or tea

Lunch

$\frac{3}{4}$ cup tomato soup
Open-face toasted cheese sandwich (1 slice whole-wheat, 1 ounce
   Cheddar cheese)
Pear or nectarine
Noncaloric drink

Snack

$\frac{1}{2}$ cup nonfat fruited yogurt with 2 tablespoons granola

Dinner

Fruit cup (strawberries, melon, kiwi, and a few grapes)
3 ounces grilled salmon
$\frac{1}{2}$ cup asparagus
$\frac{1}{2}$ cup grilled zucchini or eggplant
1-ounce roll

Open calories: It's the weekend—have a cookie for dessert or 3
cups of air-popped popcorn with a video, movie, or the big game.

1,500-CALORIE MEAL PLAN MENUS

Exchanges:
5 Meat
5 Starch/bread
3 Vegetable
Open calories: 200

4 Fruit
3 Fat
2 Milk

Day 1

Breakfast

1/3 cantaloupe
2 slices reduced-calorie whole-wheat toast (or 1 slice regular whole-
    wheat) with 2 teaspoons all-fruit spread
1 cup skim or 1 percent milk*
Coffee or tea

Lunch

1-ounce pita (4") or 1/2 6" pita stuffed with mix of 2 ounces 95% fat-
    free lunch meat (lean turkey, roast beef, chicken, or ham), 1/4
    cup nonfat cottage cheese, chopped tomatoes, lettuce, sprouts,
    grated carrots, seasoned with 1 tablespoon nonfat Italian salad
    dressing
1 small apple or 1/2 cup applesauce
Noncaloric drink

Snacks

2–3 cups air-popped popcorn (if you like, season with butter-
    flavored cooking spray and nonfat butter sprinkles)
1/4 cup dried apricots or raisins

Dinner

3 ounces fillet of grilled or baked fish
Medium (6 ounces) baked potato with 1 tablespoon nonfat sour
    cream or yogurt
1/2 cup steamed broccoli with lemon-pepper seasoning
1 cup mixed green salad with 1 tablespoon nonfat dressing
1/2 cup sliced peaches and berries

Open calories possibilities: Add a tablespoon of reduced-calorie
whipped dessert topping to your dinner peaches and berries; add a
half cup cereal to breakfast or have a whole 6" pita for lunch; increase
grilled fish to 4 ounces.

*Unless otherwise specified in the menus, milk is always skim or 1 percent. If you use 2 per-
cent or whole milk add a fat exchange.

Day 2

Breakfast

$\frac{1}{2}$ cup orange or grapefruit juice

$\frac{1}{2}$ cup dry cereal (shredded wheat, oat circles, etc.) with $\frac{1}{2}$ cup milk

1 slice wheat toast with 1 teaspoon fruit spread

Coffee or tea

Lunch

Tuna salad sandwich: 2 slices reduced-calorie wheat or rye bread, $\frac{1}{4}$ cup water-packed tuna mixed with chopped celery, dill-pickle relish, and $\frac{1}{2}$ tablespoon reduced-calorie mayonnaise

$\frac{1}{2}$ cup carrot sticks

1 small apple

Noncaloric drink

Snack

Fruit whip: Blend 1 cup strawberries or $\frac{1}{2}$ banana (4.5") with $\frac{1}{2}$ cup nonfat yogurt

Dinner

4 ounces grilled or baked chicken (skinless)

1 cup green salad with nonfat, reduced-calorie dressing

1 cup summer squash medley (sauté or roast a combination of yellow squash, zucchini, green pepper, onion, garlic in 1 teaspoon olive oil)

1-ounce hard roll

$\frac{1}{2}$ cup fresh pineapple

Open calories possibilities: Add another slice of toast to breakfast; add a spinach salad to dinner; add 6 reduced-calorie whole-wheat crackers for a snack.

Day 3

Breakfast

Orange or half a banana
1 cup oatmeal
1 cup milk
Coffee or tea

Lunch

Salad bar: 2 cups mixed vegetable salad with 2 ounces lean meat
or ½ cup low-fat cottage cheese, 1 tablespoon garbanzo beans,
1 tablespoon reduced-calorie or nonfat salad dressing
6 saltine or reduced-calorie Ritz crackers
½ cup fresh fruit from salad bar (pineapple, kiwi, apple or 1 cup
strawberries, melon)
Noncaloric drink

Snacks

2 rice cakes with 1 tablespoon peanut butter
Tangerine

Dinner

3 ounces boneless pork tenderloin medallions baked with caraway
seeds and 1 cup slivered red or green cabbage (or ½ cup sauerkraut*)
½ cup stewed apple slices with/cinnamon (no sugar added)
½ cup mashed potatoes (whipped with a little skim milk and butter sprinkles)
½ cup frozen nonfat yogurt
Noncaloric drink

Open calories possibilities: Add a slice of toast to breakfast or a 1-
ounce roll to dinner; add another piece of fruit for a snack; have a
whole banana for breakfast.

*high in salt

Day Four

Breakfast

½ grapefruit
1 bagel with 1 tablespoon reduced-fat cream cheese
1 cup milk

Lunch

1 tomato stuffed with 3 ounces chicken salad prepared with chopped celery, dill-pickle chunks, and ½ tablespoon reduced-fat mayonnaise or nonfat Italian dressing
½ cup celery and carrot sticks
¼ cup raisins
Noncaloric drink

Snacks

2 apricots or plums
1 cup milk or nonfat cocoa

Dinner

1 cup spaghetti with low-fat meat sauce (made with low-fat ground turkey, 2-ounce serving)
1 cup mixed vegetable green salad with nonfat dressing
1-ounce roll or slice of Italian bread
Noncaloric drink

Open calories possibilities: 1 tablespoon grated Parmesan cheese to top the spaghetti; add ¼ apple and 10 grapes to the chicken salad; add ½ cup frozen yogurt for dessert.

Day Five

Breakfast

1/3 melon or 1 1/4 cups watermelon
3/4 cup cornflakes or other flake cereal
1 slice of toast with 1 teaspoon fruit spread
1 cup milk
Coffee or tea

Lunch

Fast food: 6-inch turkey sub on whole-wheat roll (2 ounces turkey, lettuce, tomato, green pepper, sweet pickled peppers, onion, mustard, splash of oil and vinegar)
Small apple or orange
Noncaloric drink

Snacks

1 cup milk shake made with sugar-free mix
Orange or pear

Dinner

Shrimp creole* over 1/2 cup brown rice (3 ounces shrimp)
Steamed broccoli or carrots
1 cup mixed green salad with 1 tablespoon nonfat dressing
1 cup strawberries
Noncaloric beverage

Open calories possibilities: Add a bread exchange or another 1/2 cup rice with dinner; add 1 exchange of pretzels for a snack.

Busy today? Substitute a low-fat/low-calorie frozen dinner with similar ingredients such as those made by Healthy Choice or Lean Cuisine.

*A basic creole sauce is composed of chopped tomatoes, green peppers, and onions sautéed with a bay leaf in a little olive oil.

Day Six

Breakfast

$\frac{1}{2}$ cup orange juice

Scrambled eggs (1 yolk, 2 whites, 1 teaspoon margarine) with 1 ounce lean ham

1 slice whole-wheat toast (or 2 slices reduced-calorie whole-wheat) with 1 teaspoon jelly

Coffee or tea

Lunch

1 cup plain nonfat yogurt mixed with $\frac{1}{2}$ cup fresh fruit (peaches, apricots, berries)

1 ounce baked (no-fat) tortilla chips

Noncaloric drink

Snacks

4 Ry-Krisp crackers

1 large apple

Dinner

3 ounces chicken piccata with $\frac{1}{2}$ cup pasta

$\frac{1}{2}$ cup green beans

1 cup salad medley (chunked tomato, cucumber, peppers, and capers dressed with balsamic vinegar and dillweed)

$\frac{1}{2}$ cup sugar-free pudding or low-fat (2%) ice cream

Open calories possibilities: Increase dinner pasta to 1 cup; add a second slice of toast to breakfast; add $\frac{1}{2}$ cup fruit as an after-dinner snack.

Day Seven

Breakfast

½ cup tomato or orange juice
1 English muffin with 1 teaspoon margarine or fruit spread (or 4
    pancakes [4"] with reduced-calorie syrup using open calories)
1 cup milk or coffee-flavored nonfat yogurt
Coffee or tea

Lunch

¾ cup tomato soup
Toasted cheese sandwich (2 slices whole-wheat, 1 ounce Cheddar
    cheese)
½ cup carrot sticks
Pear or nectarine
Noncaloric drink

Snack

½ cup nonfat fruited yogurt with 2 tablespoons granola

Dinner

1 cup fruit cup (strawberries, melon, kiwi, and a few grapes)
4 ounces grilled salmon
½ cup asparagus
½ cup grilled zucchini or eggplant
1-ounce roll

Open calories possibilities: It's the weekend—have a cookie for dessert or 3 cups of air-popped popcorn with a video, movie, or the big game; stew up some apples or dried fruit to go over your breakfast pancakes.

1,800-CALORIE MEAL PLAN MENUS

Exchanges:

6 Meat

6 Starch/bread

4 Vegetable

Open calories: 300

4 Fruit

4 Fat

2 Milk

Day 1

Breakfast

$\frac{1}{3}$ cantaloupe

2 slices reduced-calorie whole-wheat toast (or 1 slice regular whole-wheat) with 2 teaspoons all-fruit spread

$\frac{1}{2}$ cup dry cereal

1 cup skim or 1 percent milk*

Coffee or tea

Lunch

1-ounce pita (4") or $\frac{1}{2}$ 6" pita stuffed with mix of 2 ounces 95% fat-free lunch meat (lean turkey, roast beef, chicken, or ham), $\frac{1}{4}$ cup nonfat cottage cheese, chopped tomatoes, lettuce, sprouts, grated carrots seasoned with 1 tablespoon nonfat Italian salad dressing

$\frac{1}{2}$ cup carrot sticks

1 small apple or $\frac{1}{2}$ cup applesauce

Noncaloric drink

Snacks

2–3 cups air-popped popcorn (if you like, season with butter-flavored cooking spray and nonfat butter sprinkles)

$\frac{1}{4}$ cup dried apricots or raisins

Dinner

4 ounces fillet of grilled or baked fish

Medium (6 ounces) baked potato with 1 tablespoon nonfat sour cream or yogurt

$\frac{1}{2}$ cup steamed broccoli with lemon-pepper seasoning

1 cup mixed green salad with 1 tablespoon nonfat dressing

$\frac{1}{2}$ cup sliced peaches and berries

Open calories possibilities: Add a tablespoon of reduced-calorie whipped dessert topping to your dinner peaches and berries or $\frac{1}{2}$ cup of frozen yogurt; have a 6" pita for lunch.

*Unless otherwise specified in the menus, milk is always skim or 1 percent. If you use 2 percent or whole milk add a fat exchange.

Day 2

Breakfast

$^{1}/_{2}$ cup orange or grapefruit juice
$^{1}/_{2}$ cup dry cereal (shredded wheat, oat circles, etc.) with $^{1}/_{2}$ cup milk
1 slice wheat toast with 1 tablespoon peanut butter
Coffee or tea

Lunch

Tuna salad sandwich: 2 slices wheat or rye bread, $^{1}/_{4}$ cup water-packed tuna mixed with chopped celery, dill-pickle relish, and $^{1}/_{2}$ tablespoon reduced-calorie mayonnaise
1 cup carrot sticks
1 small apple
Noncaloric drink

Snack

Fruit whip: Blend 1 cup strawberries or $^{1}/_{2}$ banana (4.5") with $^{1}/_{2}$ cup nonfat yogurt

Dinner

4 ounces grilled or baked chicken (skinless)
1 cup green salad with nonfat, reduced-calorie dressing
1 cup summer squash medley (sauté or roast a combination of yellow squash, zucchini, green pepper, onion, garlic in 1 teaspoon of olive oil)
1-ounce hard roll
$^{1}/_{2}$ cup fresh pineapple

Open calories possibilities: Add another slice of toast to breakfast; add a spinach salad to dinner; add 6 reduced-calorie whole-wheat crackers for a snack. Add another piece of fruit for a snack.

Day 3

Breakfast

Orange or half a banana
1 cup oatmeal
1 cup milk
Coffee or tea

Lunch

Salad bar: 3 cups mixed vegetable salad with 2 ounces lean meat
or ½ cup low-fat cottage cheese, 1 tablespoon garbanzo beans,
2 tablespoons reduced calorie or nonfat salad dressing
6 saltine or reduced-calorie Ritz crackers
½ cup fresh fruit from salad bar (pineapple, kiwi, apple or 1 cup
strawberries, melon)
Noncaloric drink

Snacks

2 rice cakes with 1 tablespoon peanut butter
Tangerine
¾ ounce low-fat cheese crackers

Dinner

4 ounces boneless pork tenderloin medallions baked with caraway
seeds and 1 cup slivered red or green cabbage (or ½ cup sauerkraut*)
½ cup stewed apple slices with cinnamon (no sugar added)
½ cup mashed potatoes (whipped with a little skim milk and butter sprinkles)
½ cup frozen nonfat yogurt
Noncaloric drink

Open calories possibilities: Add a slice of toast to breakfast or a 1-
ounce roll to dinner; add another piece of fruit for a snack; have a
whole banana for breakfast.

*high in salt

Day Four

Breakfast

$1/2$ grapefruit
1 bagel with 1 tablespoon reduced-fat cream cheese
1 cup milk

Lunch

1 tomato stuffed with 3 ounces chicken salad prepared with
    chopped celery, dill-pickle chunks, and $1/2$ tablespoon reduced
    fat mayonnaise or nonfat Italian dressing
$3/4$ ounce low-fat crackers
$1/2$ cup celery and carrot sticks
$1/4$ cup raisins
Noncaloric drink

Snacks

2 apricots or plums
1 cup milk or nonfat cocoa

Dinner

1 cup spaghetti with low-fat meat sauce (made with low-fat ground
    turkey, 3-ounce serving)
$1/2$ cup steamed broccoli or yellow squash
1 cup mixed vegetable green salad with nonfat dressing
1-ounce roll or slice of Italian bread
Noncaloric drink

Open calories possibilities: 1 tablespoon grated Parmesan cheese to
top the spaghetti; add $1/4$ apple and 10 grapes to the chicken salad; add
$1/2$ cup frozen yogurt for dessert. Add another $1/2$ cup pasta to dinner or
a snack of 2 to 3 cups plain air-popped popcorn.

Day Five

Breakfast

⅓ melon or 1¼ cups watermelon
¾ cup cornflakes or other flake cereal
1 slice of toast with 1 teaspoon fruit spread
1 cup milk
Coffee or tea

Lunch

Fast food: 6-inch turkey sub on whole-wheat roll (2 ounces turkey,
    lettuce, tomato, green pepper, sweet pickled peppers, onion,
    mustard, splash of oil and vinegar)
Small apple or orange
Noncaloric drink

Snacks

1 cup milk shake made with sugar-free mix
Orange or pear
Cucumber, pepper, and carrot slices with salsa

Dinner

Shrimp creole* over 1 cup brown rice (4 ounces shrimp)
Steamed broccoli or carrots
1 cup mixed green salad with 1 tablespoon nonfat dressing
1 cup strawberries
Noncaloric beverage

Open calories possibilities: Add a bread exchange with dinner; add
1 exchange of pretzels for a snack, or a snack of 1 exchange of crackers
and 1 ounce reduced-fat cheese.

Busy today? Substitute a low-fat/low-calorie frozen dinner with
similar ingredients such as those made by Healthy Choice or Lean
Cuisine.

*A basic creole sauce is composed of chopped tomatoes, green peppers, and onions sautéed
with a bay leaf in a little olive oil.

Day Six

Breakfast

½ cup orange juice

Scrambled eggs (1 yolk, 2 whites, 1 teaspoon margarine) with 2
    ounces lean ham

2 slices whole-wheat toast with 1 teaspoon jelly each

Coffee or tea

Lunch

1 cup plain nonfat yogurt mixed with ½ cup fresh fruit (peaches,
    apricots, berries)

1 ounce baked (no-fat) tortilla chips

Noncaloric drink

Snacks

4 Ry-Krisp crackers

1 large apple

Dinner

3 ounces chicken piccata with ½ cup pasta

½ cup green beans

½ cup cooked carrots and snow peas

1 cup salad medley (chunked tomato, cucumber, peppers, and
    capers dressed with balsamic vinegar and dill weed; include
    one fat exchange of black olives if you like)

1-ounce roll

½ cup sugar-free pudding or low-fat (2%) ice cream

Open calories possibilities: Increase dinner pasta to 1 cup; add a
snack of 2 to 3 cups air-popped popcorn. Add ½ cup fruit as an after-
dinner snack.

Day Seven

Breakfast

$^1/_2$ cup tomato or orange juice

1 English muffin with 1 teaspoon margarine or fruit spread (or 4
pancakes [4"] with reduced-calorie syrup using open calories)

1 cup milk or coffee-flavored nonfat yogurt

Coffee or tea

Lunch

$^3/_4$ cup tomato soup

Ham and cheese sandwich (2 slices whole-wheat, 1 ounce Cheddar
cheese, 1 ounce ham, mustard)

$^1/_2$ cup carrot sticks

Pear or nectarine

Noncaloric drink

Snacks

$^1/_2$ cup nonfat fruited yogurt with 2 tablespoons granola

1 exchange of pretzels or baked no-fat tortilla or potato chips with
salsa

Dinner

1 cup fruit cup (strawberries, melon, kiwi, and a few grapes)

4 ounces grilled salmon

$^1/_2$ cup asparagus

$^1/_2$ cup grilled zucchini or eggplant

1-ounce roll

Open calories: It's the weekend—have a cookie for dessert or 3
cups of air-popped popcorn with a video, movie, or the big game; stew
up some apples or dried fruit to go over your breakfast pancakes. Add
fruit as a snack.

FOOD-EXCHANGE LISTS*

The foods listed within each category have approximately the same amount of protein, fat, carbohydrate, and calories per serving. Every food is listed with a serving size that equals one exchange.

STARCH/BREAD LIST

Each item in this list contains approximately 15 grams of carbohydrates, 3 grams of protein, a trace of fat, and 80 calories. Whole-grain products average about 2 grams of fiber per exchange. Some foods are higher in fiber. Those foods that contain 3 or more grams of fiber per exchange are footnoted.

You can choose your starch exchanges from any of the items on this list. If you want to eat a starch food that is not on this list, the general rule is that:

- ¹/₂ cup of cereal, grain, or pasta is one exchange.
- 1 ounce of a bread product is one exchange.

*The exchange lists are the bases of a meal-planning system designed by a committee of the American Diabetes Association and American Dietetic Association. While designed primarily for people with diabetes and others who must follow special diets, the exchange lists are based on principles of good nutrition that apply to everyone. Copyright © 1986 American Diabetes Association, American Dietetic Association. Used by permission.

CEREALS/GRAINS/PASTA

Bran cereals,* concentrated (such as Bran Buds, All Bran)	⅓ cup
Bran cereals,* (flaked)	½ cup
Bulgur (cooked)	½ cup
Cooked cereal	½ cup
Cornmeal (dry)	2½ tbsp.
Grape-Nuts	3 tbsp.
Grits (cooked)	½ cup
Other ready-to-eat unsweetened cereals	¾ cup
Pasta (cooked)	½ cup
Puffed cereal	1½ cups
Rice, white or brown (cooked)	⅓ cup
Shredded wheat	½ cup
Wheat germ*	3 tbsp.

*3 g. or more of fiber per exchange.

DRIED BEANS/PEAS/LENTILS

Beans and peas (cooked) such as kidney, white, split, black-eyed	⅓ cup
Lentils* (cooked)	⅓ cup
Baked beans*	¼ cup

*3 g. or more of fiber per exchange.

STARCHY VEGETABLES

Corn*	½ cup
Corn on cob,* 6 in. long	1
Lima beans*	½ cup
Peas, green* (canned or frozen)	½ cup
Plantain*	½ cup
Potato, baked	1 small (3 oz)
Potato, mashed	½ cup
Squash, winter* (acorn, butternut)	¾ cup
Yam, sweet potato, plain	⅓ cup

*3 g. or more of fiber per exchange.

BREAD

Bagel	½ (1 oz)
Breadsticks, crisp, 4 in. long × ½in.	2 (⅔ oz)
Croutons, low-fat	1 cup
English muffin	½
Frankfurter or hamburger bun	½ (1 oz)
Pita, 6 in. across	½
Plain roll, small	1 (1 oz)
Raisin, unfrosted	1 slice (1 oz)
Rye, pumpernickel	1 slice (1 oz)
Tortilla, 6 in. across	1
White (including French, Italian)	1 slice (1 oz.)
Whole wheat	1 slice (1 oz.)

CRACKERS/SNACKS

Animal crackers	8
Graham crackers, 2½ in. square	3
Matzoh	¾ oz.
Melba toast	5 slices
Oyster crackers	24
Popcorn (popped, no fat added)	3 cups
Pretzels	¾ oz
Ry-Krisp,* 2 in. × 3½ in.	4
Saltine-type crackers	6
Whole wheat crackers,* no fat added (crisp breads, such as Finn, Kavli, Wasa)	2–4 slices (¾ oz.)

*3 g. or more of fiber per exchange.

STARCH FOODS PREPARED WITH FAT

Count as 1 Starch/Bread Exchange, Plus 1 Fat Exchange

Biscuit, 2½ in. across	1
Chow mein noodles	½ cup
Corn bread, 2-in. cube	1 (2 oz.)
Cracker, round butter type	6
French-fried potatoes, 2 in. to 3½ in. long	10 (1½ oz.)
Muffin, plain, small	1
Pancake, 4 in. across	2
Stuffing, bread (prepared)	¼ cup
Taco shell, 6 in. across	2
Waffle, 4½ in. square	1
Whole-wheat crackers,* fat added (such as Triscuit)	4-6 (1 oz.)

*3 g. or more of fiber per exchange.

MEAT LIST

Each serving of meat and substitutes in this list contains about 7 grams of protein. The amount of fat and number of calories vary, depending on what kind of meat or substitute you choose. The list is divided into three parts based on the amount of fat and calories: lean meat, medium-fat meat, and high-fat meat. One ounce (one meat exchange) of each of these includes:

	Carbohydrate (Grams)	Protein (Grams)	Fat (Grams)	Calories
Lean	0	7	3	55
Medium fat	0	7	5	75
High fat	0	7	8	100

You are encouraged to use lean meat, poultry, and fish in your meal plan. This will help decrease your fat intake, which may help decrease your risk of heart disease. The items from the high-fat group are high in saturated fat, cholesterol, and calories. Meat and substitutes do not contribute any fiber to your meal plan.

Meats and meat substitutes that have 400 milligrams or more of sodium per exchange are footnoted.

Meats and meat substitutes that have 400 milligrams or more of sodium if two or more exchanges are eaten are footnoted.

Tips

- Bake, roast, broil, grill, or boil these foods rather than fry them with added fat.
- Use a nonstick pan spray or a nonstick pan to brown or fry these foods.
- Trim off visible fat before and after cooking.
- Do not add flour, bread crumbs, coating mixes, or fat to these foods when preparing them.
- Weigh meat after removing bones and fat, and after cooking. Three ounces of cooked meat is about equal to 4 ounces of raw meat. Some examples of meat portions are:
  2 ounces meat (2 meat exchanges) =
    1 small chicken leg or thigh
    ½ cup cottage cheese or tuna
  3 ounces meat (3 meat exchanges) =
    1 medium pork chop

1 small hamburger
$^1/_2$ whole chicken breast
1 unbreaded fish fillet
cooked meat, about the size of a deck of cards

- Restaurants usually serve prime cuts of meat, which are high in fat and calories.

LEAN MEAT AND SUBSTITUTES

	One exchange is equal to any one of the following items:	
Beef	USDA Select or Choice grades of lean beef such as round, sirloin, and flank steak; tenderloin; and chipped beef*	1 oz.
Pork	Lean pork, such as fresh ham; canned, cured, or boiled ham,* Canadian bacon,* tenderloin	1 oz.
Veal	All cuts are lean except for veal cutlets (ground or cubed); examples of lean veal are chops and roasts	1 oz.
Poultry	Chicken, turkey, Cornish hen (without skin)	1 oz.
Fish	All fresh and frozen fish	1 oz.
	Crab, lobster, scallops, shrimp, clams (fresh or canned in water)	2 oz.
	Oysters	6 medium
	Tuna† (canned in water)	$^1/_4$ cup
	Herring† (uncreamed or smoked)	1 oz.
	Sardines (canned)	2 medium
Wild game	Venison, rabbit, squirrel	1 oz.
	Pheasant, duck, goose (without skin)	1 oz.
Cheese	Any cottage cheese†	$^1/_4$ cup
	Grated Parmesan	2 tbsp.
	Diet cheeses* (with less than 55 calories per ounce)	1 oz.
Other	95 percent fat-free luncheon meat*	1 oz.
	Egg whites	3 whites
	Egg substitutes with less than 55 calories per cup	$^1/_4$ cup

*400 mg. or more of sodium per exchange.
†400 mg. or more of sodium if two or more exchanges are eaten.

MEDIUM-FAT MEAT AND SUBSTITUTES

One exchange is equal to any one of the following items:

Beef	Most beef products fall into this category, such as all ground beef, roast (rib, chuck, rump) steak (cubed, porterhouse, T-bone), and meat loaf	1 oz.
Pork	Most pork products fall into this category, such as chops, loin roast, Boston butt and cutlets	1 oz.
Lamb	Most lamb products fall into this category, such as chops, leg, and roast	1 oz.
Veal	Cutlet (ground or cubed, unbreaded)	1 oz.
Poultry	Chicken (with skin), domestic duck or goose (well drained of fat), ground turkey	1 oz.
Fish	Tuna* (canned in oil and drained)	¼ cup
	Salmon* (canned)	¼ cup
Cheese	Skim or part-skim milk cheeses, such as	
	Ricotta	¼ cup
	Mozzarella	1 oz.
	Diet cheeses (with 56–80 calories per ounce)	1 oz.
Other	86 percent fat-free luncheon meat*	1 oz.
	Egg (high in cholesterol, limit to 3 per week)	1
	Egg substitutes with 56–80 calories per ¼ cup	¼ cup
	Tofu (2½ in. × 2¾ in. × 1 in.)	4 oz.
	Liver, heart, kidney, sweetbreads (high in cholesterol)	1 oz.

*400 mg. or more of sodium if two or more exchanges are eaten.
†400 mg. or more of sodium per exchange.

HIGH-FAT MEAT AND SUBSTITUTES

Remember, these items are high in saturated fat, cholesterol, and calories. One exchange is equal to any one of the following items.

Beef	Most USDA prime cuts of beef, such as ribs, corned beef*	1 oz.
Pork	Spareribs, ground pork, pork sausage† (patty or link)	1 oz.
Lamb	Patties (ground lamb)	1 oz.
Fish	Any fried fish product	1 oz.
Cheese	All regular cheeses, such as American,† Blue,† Cheddar,† Monterey Jack,† Swiss	1 oz.
Other	Luncheon meat such as bologna, salami, pimiento loaf†	1 oz.
	Sausage,† such as Polish, Italian smoked	1 oz.
	Knockwurst†	1 oz.
	Bratwurst*	1 oz.
	Frankfurter† (turkey or chicken)	1 frank (10/lb.)
	Peanut butter (contains unsaturated fat)	1 tbsp.
	Count as one high-fat meat plus one fat exchange	
	Frankfurter† (beef, pork, or combination)	1 frank (10/lb.)

*400 mg. or more of sodium if two or more exchanges are eaten.
†400 mg. or more of sodium per exchange.

VEGETABLE LIST

Each vegetable serving in this list contains about 5 grams of carbohydrates, 2 grams of protein, and 25 calories. Vegetables contain 2 to 3 grams of dietary fiber. Vegetables that contain 400 milligrams or more of sodium per exchange are footnoted.

Vegetables are good sources of vitamins and minerals. Fresh and frozen vegetables have more vitamins and less added salt. Rinsing canned vegetables will remove much of the salt.

Unless otherwise noted, the serving size for vegetables (one vegetable exchange) is:

- ½ cup of cooked vegetables or vegetable juice
- 1 cup of raw vegetables

Starchy vegetables, such as corn, peas, and potatoes, are in the starch/bread list.

Artichoke (½ medium)
Asparagus
Beans (green, wax, Italian)
Bean sprouts
Beets
Broccoli
Brussels sprouts
Cabbage, cooked
Carrots
Cauliflower
Eggplant
Greens (collard, mustard, turnip)
Kohlrabi
Leeks

Mushrooms, cooked
Okra
Onions
Pea pods
Peppers (green)
Rutabaga
Sauerkraut*
Spinach, cooked
Summer squash (crookneck)
Tomato (one large)
Tomato/vegetable juice*
Turnips
Water chestnuts
Zucchini, cooked

*400 mg. or more of sodium per exchange.

FRUIT LIST

Each item in the following list contains about 15 grams of carbohydrates and 60 calories. Fresh, frozen, and dried fruits have about 2 grams of fiber per exchange. Fruits that have 3 or more grams of fiber per exchange are footnoted.

The carbohydrate and calorie contents for a fruit exchange are based on the usual serving of the most commonly eaten fruits. Use fresh fruits or fruits frozen or canned without sugar added. Whole fruit is more filling than fruit juice and may be a better choice for those who are trying to lose weight. Unless otherwise noted, the serving size for one fruit exchange is:

- ½ cup of fresh fruit or fruit juice
- ¼ cup of dried fruit

FRESH, FROZEN, AND UNSWEETENED CANNED FRUIT

Apple (raw, 2 in. across)	1 apple
Applesauce (unsweetened)	½ cup
Apricots (medium, raw)	4 apricots
Apricots (canned)	½ cup, or 4 halves
Banana (9 in. long)	½ banana
Blackberries* (raw)	¾ cup
Blueberries* (raw)	¾ cup
Cantaloupe (5 in. across)	⅓ melon
(cubes)	1 cup
Cherries (large, raw)	12 cherries
Cherries (canned)	½ cup
Figs (raw, 2 in. across)	2 figs
Fruit cocktail (canned)	½ cup
Grapefruit (medium)	½ grapefruit
Grapefruit (segments)	¾ cup
Grapes (small)	15 grapes
Honeydew melon (medium)	⅛ melon
(cubes)	1 cup
Kiwi (large)	1 kiwi
Mandarin oranges	¾ cup
Mango (small)	½ mango
Nectarine* (2½ in. across)	1 nectarine
Orange (2½ in. across)	1 orange
Papaya	1 cup
Peach (2¾ in. across)	1 peach, or ¾ cup
Peaches (canned)	½ cup, or 2 halves
Pear	½ large, or 1 small
Pears (canned)	½ cup, or 2 halves
Persimmon (medium, native)	2 persimmons
Pineapple (raw)	¾ cup
Pineapple (canned)	⅓ cup
Plum (raw 2 in. across)	2 plums
Pomegranate*	½ pomegranate
Raspberries* (raw)	1 cup
Strawberries* (raw whole)	1¼ cups
Tangerine* (2½ in. across)	2 tangerines
Watermelon (cubes)	1¼ cups

*3 g. or more of fiber per exchange.

DRIED FRUIT

Apples*	4 rings
Apricots*	7 halves
Dates	2½ medium
Figs*	1½
Prunes*	3 medium
Raisins	2 tbsp.

*3 g. or more of fiber per exchange

FRUIT JUICE

Apple juice/cider	½ cup
Cranberry juice cocktail	⅓ cup
Grapefruit juice	½ cup
Grape juice	⅓ cup
Orange juice	½ cup
Pineapple juice	½ cup
Prune juice	⅓ cup

MILK LIST

Each serving of milk or milk products in this list contains about 12 grams of carbohydrates and 8 grams of protein. The amount of fat in milk is measured in percent of butterfat. The calories vary, depending on what kind of milk you choose. The list is divided into three parts, based on the amount of fat and calories: skim/very low-fat milk, low-fat milk, and whole milk. One serving (one milk exchange) of each of these includes:

	Carbohydrate (Grams)	Protein (Grams)	Fat (Grams)	Calories
Skim/very low-fat	12	8	trace	90
Low-fat	12	8	5	120
Whole	12	8	8	150

Milk is the body's main source of calcium, the mineral needed for growth and repair of bones. Yogurt is also a good source of calcium. Yogurt and many dry or powdered milk products have different amounts of fat. If you have questions about a particular item, read the label to find out the fat and calorie content.

Milk is good to drink, and it can be added to cereal and to other foods.

SKIM AND VERY LOW-FAT MILK

Skim milk	1 cup
½ percent milk	1 cup
1 percent milk	1 cup
Low-fat buttermilk	1 cup
Evaporated skim milk	½ cup
Dry nonfat milk	⅓ cup
Plain nonfat yogurt	8 oz.

LOW-FAT MILK

2 percent milk	1 cup fluid
Plain low-fat yogurt (with added nonfat milk solids)	8 oz.

WHOLE MILK

The whole milk group has much more fat per serving than the skim and low-fat groups. Whole milk has more than 3¼ percent butterfat. Try to limit your choices from the whole milk group as much as possible.

Whole milk	1 cup
Evaporated whole milk	½ cup
Whole plain yogurt	8 oz.

FAT LIST

Each serving in this list contains about 5 grams of fat and 45 calories.

The foods in this list contain mostly fat, although some items may also contain a small amount of protein. All fats are high in calories and should be carefully measured. Everyone should modify fat intake by eating unsaturated fats instead of saturated fats.

UNSATURATED FATS

Avocado	⅛ medium
Margarine	1 tsp.
Margarine*, diet	1 tbsp.
Mayonnaise	1 tsp.

Mayonnaise*, reduced-calorie	1 tbsp.
Nuts and seeds:	
Almonds, dry roasted	6 whole
Cashews, dry roasted	1 tbsp.
Pecans	2 whole
Peanuts	20 small or 10 large
Walnuts	2 whole
Other nuts	1 tbsp.
Seeds, pine nuts, sunflower (without shells)	1 tbsp.
Pumpkin seeds	2 tsp.
Oil (corn, cottonseed, safflower, soybean, sunflower, olive, peanut)	1 tsp.
Olives*	10 small or 5 large
Salad dressing, mayonnaise type	2 tsp.
Salad dressing, mayonnaise type, reduced calorie	1 tbsp.
Salad dressing* (oil varieties)	1 tbsp.
Salad dressing,† reduced calorie	2 tbsp.

*400 mg. or more of sodium if two or more exchanges are eaten.
†400 mg. or more of sodium per exchange.

SATURATED FATS

Butter	1 tsp.
Bacon*	1 slice
Chitterlings	½ ounce
Coconut, shredded	2 tbsp.
Coffee whitener, liquid	2 tbsp.
Coffee whitener, powder	4 tsp.
Cream (light, coffee, table)	2 tbsp.
Cream, sour	2 tbsp.
Cream (heavy, whipping)	1 tbsp.
Cream cheese	1 tbsp.
Salt pork*	¼ ounce

*400 mg. or more of sodium if two or more exchanges are eaten.

FREE FOODS

A free food is any food or drink that contains less than 20 calories per serving. You can eat as much as you want of those items that have no serving size specified. You may eat two or three servings per day of those items that have a specific serving size. Be sure to spread them out through the day.

DRINKS

Bouillon, or broth without fat*	Cocoa powder, unsweetened (1 tbsp.)
Bouillon, low-sodium	Coffee/tea
Carbonated drinks, sugar-free	Drink mixes, sugar-free
Carbonated water	Tonic water, sugar-free
Club soda	

*400 mg. or more of sodium per exchange.

NONSTICK PAN SPRAY

FRUIT

Cranberries, unsweetened (½ cup)	Rhubarb, unsweetened (½ cup)

VEGETABLES (RAW, 1 CUP)

Cabbage	Hot peppers
Celery	Mushrooms
Chinese cabbage*	Radishes
Cucumber	Zucchini*
Green onion	

*3 g. or more of fiber per exchange.

SALAD GREENS

Endive	Romaine
Escarole	Spinach
Lettuce	

SWEET SUBSTITUTES

Candy, hard, sugar-free	Pancake syrup, sugar-free (1–2 tbsp.)
Gelatin, sugar-free	Sugar substitutes (saccharin,
Gum, sugar-free	Aspartame)
Jam/jelly, sugar-free	Whipped topping (2 tbsp.)
(less than 20 cal./2 tsp.)	

CONDIMENTS

Ketchup (1 tbsp.)	Salad dressing,† low-calorie (2 tbsp.)
Horseradish	Taco sauce (1 tbsp.)
Mustard	Vinegar
Pickles,* dill, unsweetened	

*400 mg. or more of sodium per exchange.
†The nutritionists who developed the diet for The Rockport Walking Program suggest that only those salad dressings with 10 calories or less per tablespoon be considered "free foods."

Seasonings (see the following material) can be very helpful in making food taste better. Be careful of how much sodium you use. Read the label, and choose those seasonings that do not contain sodium or salt.

SEASONINGS

Basil (fresh)	Lemon pepper
Celery seeds	Lime
Chili powder	Lime juice
Chives	Mint
Cinnamon	Onion powder
Curry	Oregano
Dill	Paprika
Flavoring extracts (vanilla,	Pepper
almond, walnut, peppermint,	Pimiento
butter, lemon, etc.)	Spices
Garlic	Soy sauce*
Garlic powder	Soy sauce,* low-sodium ("lite")
Herbs	Wine, used in cooking (¼ cup)
Hot pepper sauce	Worcestershire sauce
Lemon	
Lemon juice	

*400 mg. or more of sodium per exchange.

COMBINATION FOODS

Much of the food we eat is mixed in various combinations. These combination foods do not fit into only one exchange list. It can be quite hard to tell what is in a certain casserole dish or baked food item. This is a list of average values for some typical combination foods. This list will help you fit these foods into your meal plans.

Food	Amount	Exchanges
Casseroles, homemade	1 cup (8 oz.)	2 starch, 2 medium-fat meat, 1 fat
Cheese pizza,* thin crust	¼ of 15 oz., or ¼ of 10 in.	2 starch, 1 medium-fat meat, 1 fat
Chili with beans*† (commercial)	1 cup (8 oz.)	2 starch, 2 medium-fat meat, 2 fat
Chow mein* (without noodles or rice)	2 cups (16 oz.)	1 starch, 2 vegetable, 2 lean meat
Macaroni and cheese*	1 cup (8 oz.)	2 starch, 1 medium-fat meat, 2 fat
Soup		
Bean*†	1 cup (8 oz.)	1 starch, 1 vegetable, 1 lean meat
Chunky, all varieties*	10¾ oz. can	1 starch, 1 vegetable, 1 medium-fat meat
Cream* (made with water)	1 cup (8 oz.)	1 starch, 1 fat
Vegetable* or broth type*	1 cup (8 oz.)	1 starch
Spaghetti and meatballs* (canned)	1 cup (8 oz.)	2 starch, 1 medium-fat meat, 1 fat
If beans are used as a meat substitute		
Dried beans,† peas,† lentils	1 cup (cooked)	2 starch, 1 lean meat

*400 mg. or more of sodium per exchange.
†3 g. or more of fiber per exchange.

ADDITIONAL EXCHANGE LIST*

Starch/Bread list		
Bread, low-calorie (40 calories per slice)	2 slices	
Bread crumbs, dried	3 tbsp.	
Rice cakes	2	
Zwieback cookies	2	
Arrowroot cookies	4	
Vanilla wafers	5	
Gingersnaps	3	
Flour	3 tbsp.	
Cornstarch	3 tbsp.	
Low-fat cookies	¾ oz.	
Vegetable List		
Mixed vegetables (frozen)	⅓ cup	
Peas and carrots (frozen)	⅓ cup	
Fat list		
Tartar sauce	2 tsp.	
Milk list		
Sugar-free hot cocoa (40 calories)	2 packets	
Sugar-free pudding made with skim milk	½ cup	
Sugar-free shake mix (70 calories)	1 packet	
Fruited yogurt, nonfat, any flavor	½ cup	
Frozen yogurt, low-fat, any flavor	½ cup	
Frozen yogurt bar, low-fat	1 bar	
Fudge bar, Fudgsicle, etc. †	1 bar	
Ice milk (no more than 110 calories per serving)	½ cup	
Additional Combination Foods		
Refried beans	⅓ cup	1 starch, 1 fat
Fruited yogurt, any flavor, low-fat	1 cup	1 milk, 2 fruit, ½ fat
Granola	¼ cup	1 starch, 1 fat
Granola bar	1 small	1 starch, 1 fat
Snack chips	1 ounce	1 starch, 2 fat
Microwave popcorn	3½ cups (or ⅓ of a 10-cup bag)	1 starch, 1 fat

*Adapted with permission from *The Rockport Walking Program* (New York: Prentice Hall, 1989).
†There are many low-calorie frozen desserts on the market today. Many of them are made with low-fat milk and have less than 100 calories. These may be included in the diet and counted as one milk exchange.

ADDITIONAL FREE FOODS*

Seasonings

Flavored crystals
  (Butter Buds, Molly McButter, etc.)
Crystal Light Bars (14 calories/bar)
Tabasco
Salsa
Teriyaki
Salt
Celery salt
Garlic salt
Onion salt
All spices and herbs
Ginger, fresh or powder
Tenderizers
No-oil salad dressing

*Adapted with permission from *The Rockport Walking Program* (New York: Prentice Hall, 1989).

ALCOHOL

We've designed the eating program to be a practical, flexible plan that you'll want to stick with for the long term. And because we recognize that having a glass of wine or a beer with dinner is appropriate for many people, we're including information on alcoholic beverages in reasonable amounts.

We stress moderation here, not only because of the obvious physical and psychological dangers of too much alcohol but also because alcohol provides calories and not much else in the way of nutrition. And with 7 calories per gram, alcohol nearly matches fat's 9 calories per gram.

Type	Amount	Exchange
Table Wine	4 oz.	2 fats
Beer	12 oz.	1 starch, 2 fats
Beer, light	12 oz.	2 fats
Whiskey, gin, vodka, scotch, etc.	1.5 oz. (1 shot)	2 fats

SELECTED REFERENCES

1. Damitz, S., Price, J., Freedson, P., Kline, G., Fletcher, E., Kreidieh, I., Rippe, J. "Determinants of Aerobic Capacity in Men and Women Ages 40–79 Years." *Med. Sci. Sports Exerc.* 1995; 27(5):S1337.

2. Price, J., Damitz, S., Palmer, C., Kreidieh, I., Freedson, P., Rippe, J. "Determinants of 50-Foot Walk Time in Older Individuals." *Med. Sci. Sports Exerc.* 1995; 27(5): S1342.

3. Kreidieh, I., Freedson, P., Kline, G., DeRuisseau, K., Hess, S., Palmer, C., DeMers, K., Rippe, J. "Gender and Age Difference in Walk Time, Reaction Time and Balance Among Individuals ages 40–79." *The Gerontologist* 1995; 35(I):77P.

4. Kreidieh, I., Freedson, P., Kline, G., Palmer, C., Damitz, S., Hess, S., Rippe, J. "Prediction of Maximum Oxygen Consumption Using 1-Mile Walk Times in Individuals Aged 40–79 Years." *Circulation* 1995; 92(8): S1–3540.

5. Rippe, J., Hess, S., Palmer, C., DeMers, K., Kreidieh, I., Kline, G., Freedson, P., "Is Physical Activity Related to VO^2max in a 40–79-Year-Old Population?" *Med. Sci. Sports Exerc.* 1996; 28(5).

6. Palmer, C., Hess, S., DeMers, K., DeRuisseau, K., Kline, G., Freedson, P., Rippe, J. "Physical Activity, and Muscular Strength and Endurance in the 40–79-Year-Old Population." (Presented, International Conference on Aging and Physical Activity, 1995).

7. Hess, S., Freedson, P., Kline, G., DeMers, K., DeRuisseau, K., Palmer, C., Kreidieh, I., Damitz, S., Rippe, J. "Aerobic Capacity, Muscular Strength and Endurance, and Flexibility Among Individuals Ages 40–79." *The Gerontologist* 1995; 35(I):109P.

8. Palmer, C., Freedson, P., Kline, G., Kreidieh, I., Hess, S., Rippe, J. "Is Balance Associated with Physical Activity, Leg Strength and Body Mass Index in an Older Population?" *The Gerontologist* 1995; 35(I):76P.

9. Rippe, J., Ward, A., Porcari, J., Freedson, P. "Walking for Health and Fitness." *JAMA* 1988; 259:2720.

10. Blair, S., Kohl, H., Paffenbarger, R., Clark, D., Cooper, K., Gibbons, L. "Physical Fitness and All-Cause Mortality: A Prospective Study of Healthy Men and Women." *JAMA* 1989; 262:2395–2401.

11. Powell, K., Thompson, P., Casperson, C., Kendrick, J. "Physical Activity and the Incidence of Coronary Heart Disease." *Ann. Rev. Publ. Health* 1987: 253–287.

12. Rippe, J. *Fit for Success: Proven Strategies for Executive Health*. New York: Prentice Hall Press, 1989.

13. Rippe, J., Price, J., DeMers, K., Damitz, S., Ahlquist, L. "The Effects of a 12-Week Hypocaloric Diet and Exercise Program on Body Composition and Cardiovascular Function in Moderately Overweight Women." *J. Gen. Int. Med.* 1995; 10(7):417.

14. Price, J., Rippe, J., DeMers, K., Damitz, S., Ahlquist, L. "The Effects of a 12-Week Diet and Exercise Program on Quality of Life in Moderately Overweight Women." *J. Gen. Int. Med.* 1995; 10(4):103.

15. Rippe, J. *Exercise Exchange Program*. New York: Simon & Schuster, 1992.

16. Rippe, J. "Staying Loose." *Modern Maturity* June–July 1990; 72–77.

17. Pate, R., Pratt, M., Blair, S., Haskell, W., Macera, C., Bouchard, C., Buckner, D., Casperson, C., Ettinger, W., Heath, G., King, A., Kriska, A., Leon, A., Marcus, B., Morris, J., Paffenbarger, R., Patrick, K., Pollack, M., Rippe, J., Sallis, J., Wilmore, J. "Physical Activity and Public Health: A Recommendation from the Centers for Disease Control and Prevention, and the American College of Sports Medicine." *JAMA* 1995; 273:402–407.

18. Hess, S., DeMers, K., Damitz, S., Wang, Y., Rippe, J. "The Effects of Heart Rate Biofeedback on Psychophysiological Responses in Anxious 40–59-Year-Old Women." *Med. Exer. Nutr. Health* 1995; 4:369–379.

19. Rippe, J. *Fit with the Advil 40+ Fit over 40 Standards*. 1995. (Available through the Advil Forum on Health Education, 1500 Broadway, 26th Floor, New York., N.Y. 10036.)

20. American College of Sports Medicine Position Stand: "The Recommended Quantity and Quality of Exercise for Developing and Maintaining Cardiorespiratory and Muscular Fitness in Healthy Adults." *Med. Sci. Sport Exerc.* 1990; 22:265–274.

21. *The Nolan Ryan Fitness Guide: Advil Forum on Health Education*. The President's Council on Physical Fitness and Sports, 1994.

22. Rippe, J. "How Hard Do You Really Need to Exercise?" *Tufts University Diet and Nutrition Letter* 1995; 13(5):4–6.

23. Brown, D., Wang, Y., Ward, A., Ebbeling, C., Fortlage, L., Puleo, E., Benson, H., Rippe, J. "Chronic Psychological Effects of Exercise and Exercise Plus Cognitive Strategies." *Med. Sci. Sports Exer.* 1995; 27:765–775.

24. Ward, A., Malloy, P., Rippe, J. "Exercise Prescription Guidelines for Normal and Cardiac Populations." *Cardiol. Clin.* 1987; 5:197–210.

25. *Polar "Take Ten" Stress Reduction Program*. New York: Polar Electro, Inc., 1995.

INDEX

Numbers in *italics* indicate charts and illustrations.